the 4-PHASE
HISTAMINE RESET PLAN

Getting to the Root of Migraines, Eczema, Vertigo, Allergies and More

DR. BECKY CAMPBELL

author of *The 30-Day Thyroid Reset Plan*

PAGE STREET
PUBLISHING CO.

PAGE STREET
PUBLISHING CO.

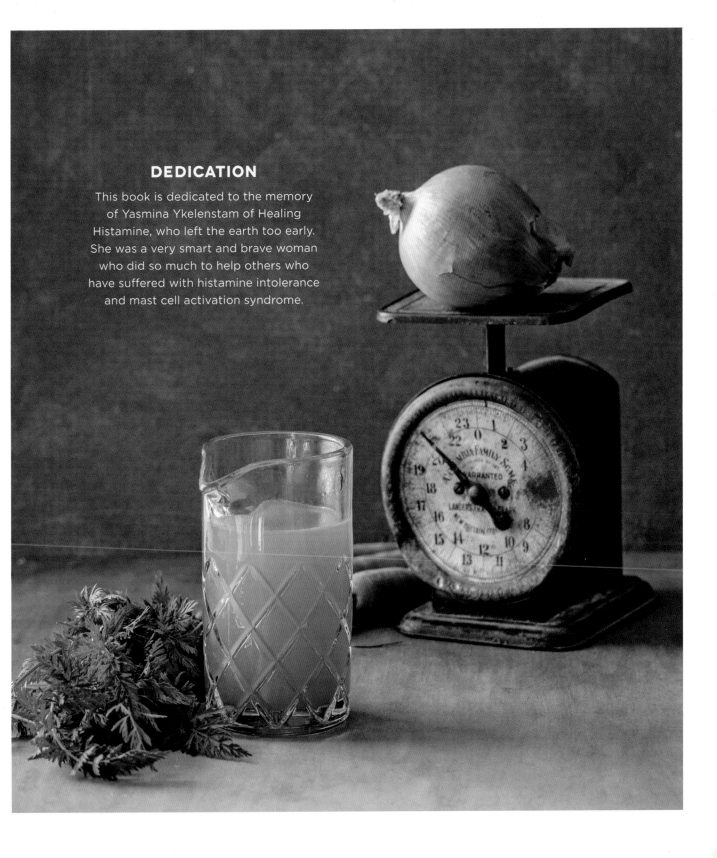

DEDICATION

This book is dedicated to the memory of Yasmina Ykelenstam of Healing Histamine, who left the earth too early. She was a very smart and brave woman who did so much to help others who have suffered with histamine intolerance and mast cell activation syndrome.

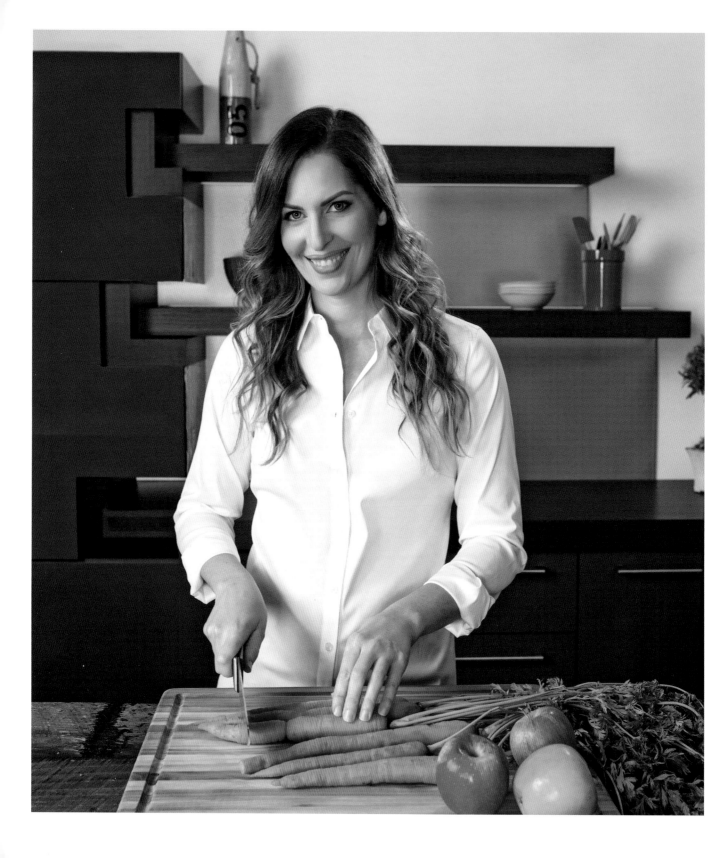

Contents

FOREWORD

At first, it's a nuisance. You try to ignore it. "It's just a headache." Again. It doesn't justify your time to dive into why it's there. It definitely doesn't justify a visit to the doctor.

Then you start experiencing another symptom on top of your headaches: "I can't fall asleep." It's not just a one-time thing. It's happening more and more, but so randomly you cannot determine the cause at all.

A few months later, you realize . . . "My eczema is flaring up." Along with . . . "These mosquito bites itch like crazy."

A year goes by and you find yourself exclaiming to a friend, "Why can't I enjoy drinking one single glass of wine?! I feel awful when I do!" Amazingly, your friend says they're struggling with exactly the same things! They are as lost as you are.

You're finally at your wit's end and off to the doctor you go.

How'd that work out? You try another one. And another one. From steroids to antibiotics. To steroids AND antibiotics. No relief. In fact, you're worse.

You learn about integrative medicine and try a naturopathic doctor. No luck. You try a functional medicine doctor. No luck. You try acupuncture. No luck. You try everything from probiotics to fish oil and vitamin D to a multivitamin. Your shelves are looking like you could run a pharmacy. You're a bit better, but still struggling.

Frustrated with all the doctors, you turn to social media forums. Perhaps that is how you found out about this book. Let me tell you right now that you're in good hands! If you're on the fence about buying it, buy it. I was just like you are right now: I had a plethora of oddball, seemingly disparate symptoms appearing randomly that did not necessitate a trip to the doctor but that certainly affected the quality of my life. Welcome to what seems like one of the fastest growing undiagnosed problems today: histamine intolerance.

Did you know that it takes on average about ten years for someone to get diagnosed with histamine intolerance?! For me, it took about thirty-five years. My histamine intolerance symptoms included:

- Bloody noses
- Irritability
- Difficulty falling asleep
- Headaches
- Eczema
- Sweaty feet (gross)
- Profuse sweating when exercising (you didn't want to guard me in basketball)
- Fast resting heart rate (about 70, even when I was fit; now it's 48)
- Super itchy mosquito bites
- Red spots all over my hands when exposed to dust mites
- Always hot

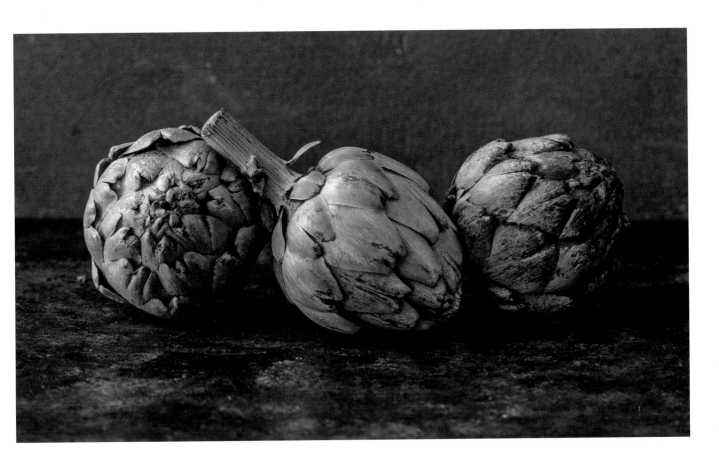

These symptoms all disappeared—that's the awesome news! The bad news? They can come roaring back quite fast, and sometimes they do. But I now know that I am genetically susceptible to histamine intolerance, and I understand why my histamine levels increase and what to do about it, so I can get myself back on track.

You can't fix what you don't know is broken. But with Dr. Campbell's book in your hands, you'll discover all things relating to histamine intolerance. It will be a lot of work. There is no quick fix here. It's up to you to implement what you read in these pages. Trust the process and stick with it. You absolutely will experience a life without histamine intolerance! Dr. Campbell will share with you a few of her tricks and she'll share a few of mine. Together, we have your back!

—DR. BEN LYNCH

Founder and president of Seeking Health,
www.seekinghealth.com

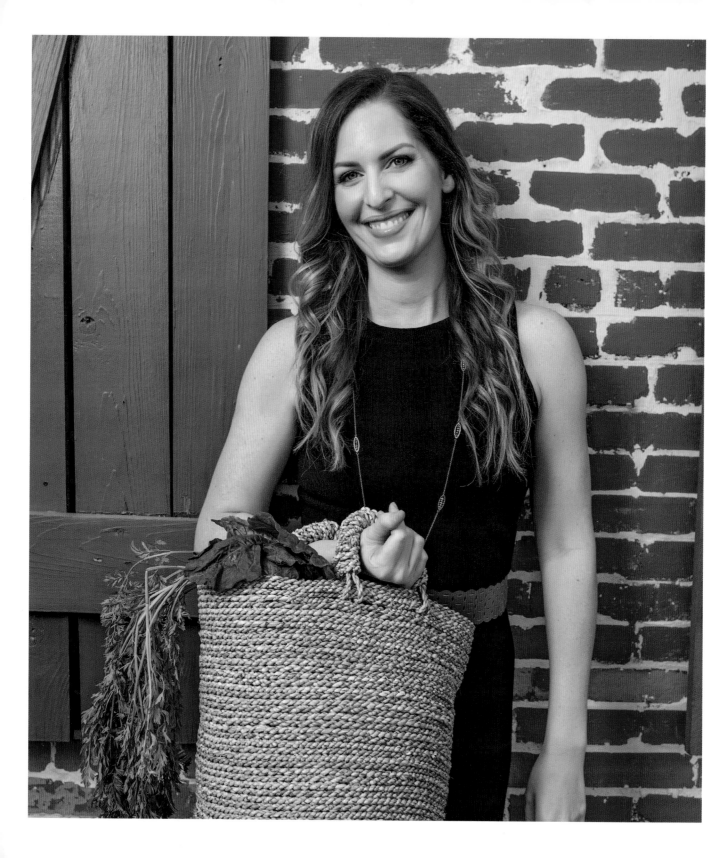

INTRODUCTION

MY STORY WITH HISTAMINE INTOLERANCE

As we start this journey together, I want you to know that this topic is personal to me in the same way it may be to you.

Those of you who know a little bit about my story from my first book, *The 30-Day Thyroid Reset Plan*, will remember that for many years, I suffered from thyroid issues that were driven by gut problems, heavy metals and viruses. But what most people don't know is that one of the most significant issues—in addition to my thyroid symptoms and my general ill health—was mast cell activation syndrome (MCAS) and, therefore, histamine intolerance. As you will learn in this book, mast cells (white blood cells) are responsible for releasing histamine. This is not a bad thing unless your body isn't equipped to break down the histamine properly or you are producing more histamine than your body can handle, which happens to be the case with MCAS.

As a kid, I had terrible heat intolerance. I would often faint in the sun, and I'd get hives out of the blue. When I ate certain foods that contain high levels of histamine, like aged meats, pickles, aged cheeses, citrus fruits and more that we will cover in this book, my scalp would tingle and a heavy fatigue would wash over me. Later, I also experienced gradually worsening symptoms like migraines, vertigo, heart palpitations, anxiety and panic attacks, acid reflux, a skin condition called seborrheic dermatitis and low blood pressure. Those symptoms never went away.

In fact, in my early twenties, when the thyroid and gut issues were at their worst, almost any food I ate caused my body to react in a negative way. Yet a histamine intolerance diagnosis was still almost a decade away.

Luckily, my situation improved a great deal when I was diagnosed with hypothyroidism, excess cortisol levels and gut issues like leaky gut, candida and parasites. Thanks to functional medicine, I was able to heal my gut and balance my thyroid and adrenal hormones, as well as eat a much wider variety of foods. However, I still experienced strange symptoms, like migraines, that no one would be able to explain for years.

It wasn't until I was 32 and began learning about histamine intolerance as a functional-medicine practitioner that I finally began to piece together the puzzle. That led to a life-changing diagnosis: I realized that my symptoms and food sensitivities were being driven by histamine intolerance brought on by some genetic mutations, like methylenetetrahydrofolate reductase (MTHFR), methylation issues and other underlying causes that we will discuss in this book. From there, I began following the plan outlined in this book, continuing to work on my health, and now I'm able to eat most foods without any problems at all. Most of the symptoms I suffered are gone and I live a pretty normal life day-to-day.

During this journey together, you'll discover which foods may be causing issues for your body, so you can also reduce the list of foods to avoid to just a handful and experience relief from the puzzling and debilitating symptoms of histamine intolerance. You will also learn what may be driving your issues with histamine and how to support your body through my four-phase plan.

I see many patients with histamine intolerance that presents itself in many different ways. I am going to share with you three patient stories so that you can see how histamine intolerance can look different for different individuals.

PATIENT STORIES

JAMES, 34

When I first met James, he was suffering from twenty-three migraines per month. James had been to see multiple migraine specialists. They had prescribed migraine medications, such as topiramate and sumatriptan. Unfortunately, they didn't help him. In fact, James was still suffering so much that he was taking approximately four ibuprofen tablets once or twice every day to somehow deal with the pain. James also complained of feeling very fatigued after he ate certain foods but was struggling to pinpoint which foods were affecting him.

I immediately suspected histamine intolerance, so I put him on a strict low-histamine diet for 30 days. We also supported his liver with the Optimal Reset Liver Love supplement. In addition, I recommended he take a histamine-supporting supplement called Histo Relief while we did some testing to look for the underlying triggers of his histamine intolerance (we'll talk about these products in later chapters).

James reacted well to the changes. His headaches decreased by 75 percent within the first two weeks and the fatigue he had been experiencing was completely gone thanks to the dietary adjustments.

When the testing came back, we also discovered that he had small intestinal bacterial overgrowth (SIBO). We worked on that with antimicrobial supplements for 60 days. Afterward, he was able to start introducing more high-histamine and histamine-liberating foods back into his diet with no ill effects.

James still has to stay away from a few foods that are high in histamine, such as aged meats and fermented foods, but he's happy to follow a mostly Paleo diet and is feeling a lot better, with no need to take any medication and few to no migraines per month.

JAN, 48

Jan came to see me complaining of fatigue and dizziness, as well as eczema all over her body and especially on the bottoms of her feet. The eczema made it hard for her to walk and do little things that most of us take for granted on a day-to-day basis. She had been put on steroids multiple times to help with the eczema but experienced little to no relief.

What Jan didn't know is that each time she took the steroids, her cortisol (stress hormone) levels were going higher and higher. This was when her fatigue really started to become a problem. She also noticed she was gaining weight in her belly with no diet change to induce it.

Because I had struggled with a skin issue (seborrheic dermatitis) related to histamine intolerance myself and had seen many other patients have the same reaction, I knew histamine intolerance was most likely at the root of her symptoms. I started Jan on a strict version of the low-histamine diet (only foods on the Yes List, page 57), because we needed to calm her system down quickly. The next thing I did was support her liver. I do this with all patients, because the liver has such a vital job, but with Jan, this was even more important. If your liver is not effectively eliminating toxins from your body, your skin will. This is common in people with skin issues like eczema, psoriasis and more.

I knew that long-term liver support was going to be vital to Jan's treatment plan in addition to the strict elimination of high-histamine foods. Once I received Jan's test results, I learned that she had leaky gut, parasites and SIBO. I have to say, I was not at all surprised with these results. She also had very high levels of cortisol that I believed were causing her fatigue and weight gain.

We worked on Jan's gut with 90 days of antimicrobial supplements followed by months of gut-lining support (Ultimate Gut Support). She eventually was able to add the foods on the Maybe List (page 57) and even some foods from the No List (page 57). In addition to these changes, Jan had to work on reducing her stress levels. I walked her through some of the techniques I will detail for you in this book. I believe managing stress and mind-set is one of the most important techniques to healing your body.

JENNIFER, 39

Jennifer came to me complaining of heart palpitations, vertigo, hives that would pop up out of the blue and a feeling of throat swelling when eating certain foods that she couldn't always pinpoint. She also said that it felt like something was crawling on her skin sometimes, which, having had this myself, I can say is a little scary.

Not only did I suspect that Jennifer had histamine intolerance, but I also suspected that her histamine intolerance was being driven by MCAS. One of the biggest reasons I suspected this was because she had had these symptoms for as long as she could remember, which is usually a big giveaway that we are dealing with MCAS (we will dive into this much deeper later in the book). With histamine intolerance, there are usually a handful of triggers, but with MCAS there are more than 200 triggers, so it can be a lot tougher to navigate what the main underlying causes are.

Jennifer also had an intolerance to extreme weather (heat or cold), which is also a significant clue that we are dealing with MCAS. For Jennifer, I had to do a little more detailed testing right out of the gate. In addition to instituting a low-histamine diet and testing her gut and hormone levels, I also wanted to see whether Jennifer had any chronic viruses or heavy metal toxicity and whether there was a possibility she had mold in her house or work environment.

It turned out that she had all of these things working against her, and this is why she was having such a severe reaction. It took a little longer to get Jennifer stable than the other two patients we have talked about, but she did become well and is stable now. This is why I go into such detail in this book about the major things to look for if a low-histamine diet doesn't resolve the majority of your symptoms.

Dr. Becky Campbell

One

AN INTRODUCTION TO HISTAMINE **AND HISTAMINE INTOLERANCE**

WHAT IS HISTAMINE?

Histamine is a chemical your body makes that plays a number of different roles, but its main function is to help your body get rid of allergens. It makes up part of the body's defense system. You have likely heard histamine mentioned before in relation to allergies and allergic reactions. You may have also taken an antihistamine at some point in your life. Medications like Benadryl, Zyrtec, Claritin or Allegra are common allergy remedies for seasonal allergy-symptom relief.

When you are suffering from seasonal allergies, the symptoms are coming from an inflammatory response stemming from the histamine release. Yet when histamine is released, it causes inflammation to alert the body of potential pathogens. In fact, histamine allows our white blood cells to find and attack pathogens, viruses and allergies by causing the blood vessels to swell. When you're not histamine intolerant, this is a natural part of the body's immune response, and enzymes later break down the histamine to prevent it from building up and causing ill health.

Histamine is also involved in digestion through stomach acid as well as the central nervous system, where it works as a neurotransmitter delivering messages between the body and the brain. In the body, histamine is produced by various immune cells, including basophils, eosinophils and mast cells. It is also found in food in the form of an amino acid called histidine, which is most commonly present in fermented foods.

WHEN HISTAMINE BECOMES A PROBLEM

Histamine can become an issue when it builds up. This can occur when the body is suffering from metabolic disturbances, such as a defect in enzyme-producing genes, that make it difficult for the body to break down and metabolize histamine in the proper way. When this happens, histamine can affect many different areas, including the brain, gut, lungs and cardiovascular system, causing a number of unwanted symptoms.

HISTAMINE

RECEPTORS IN THE BODY

HISTAMINE

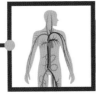

The Immune System (H1 Receptor)

Histamine functions as a vasodilator (dilates blood vessels).

The Stomach (H2 Receptor)

Histamine contorts the function of hydrochloric acid (helps with digestion).

The Brain (H3 Receptor)

Histamine acts as a neurotransmitter, moving messages about sleep, appetite, and behavior all over the brain (this is a good thing).

Bone Marrow & WBC (H4 Receptor)

These receptors are also found in the colon, liver, lung, small intestine, spleen, testes, thymus, tonsils and trachea.

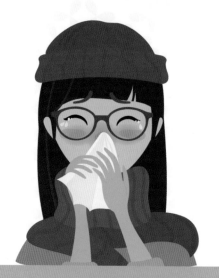

HISTAMINE

BREAKDOWN

DAO

HNMT

Histamine can be broken down by diamine oxidase (DAO) or by histamine N-menthyltransferase (HNMT).

THE KEY ROLE OF ENZYMES

There are different enzymes specific to different areas of the body that work to break down histamine. For example, histamine can be broken down by diamine oxidase (DAO) in various areas of the digestive system. DAO is a huge part of histamine metabolism, and it helps balance proper histamine levels in the body.

When in the spine, kidneys, liver, lungs and some other areas, histamine is broken down by histamine N-methyltransferase (HNMT). HNMT can break down histamine only when the histamine is in the spaces between cells, but it helps mop up excess histamine very effectively wherever it is found.

When these enzymes aren't present or when you are suffering from a metabolic issue that makes it hard to break down histamine, histamine builds up, leading to histamine intolerance and a cascade of symptoms.

HISTAMINE INTOLERANCE AND ITS SYMPTOMS

Histamine intolerance is not a sensitivity to histamine as you might imagine, but an indication that too much of it has built up in the body or that there is an inability to break it down properly. Histamine intolerance is becoming more common due to more recognition, more medications being taken that inactivate the enzymes responsible for histamine breakdown, more gut issues coming from the use of antibiotics and chemicals in foods and other reasons. Many of my patients suffer from it, as do I, which has allowed me to develop an in-depth understanding of its symptoms and the damage it can do to your health.

The symptoms of histamine intolerance are quite similar to symptoms of seasonal allergies, but some symptoms can be much more severe. They include the following:

- Itchy skin, eyes, ears and nose
- Eczema or other types of dermatitis
- Red eyes
- Hives
- Facial swelling or other tissue swelling
- Tightness in the throat
- Difficulty regulating body temperature
- A drop in blood pressure when standing up quickly
- Vertigo or dizziness (see sidebar, page 17)
- Low blood pressure
- Fast heart rate
- Heart palpitations
- Difficulty falling asleep
- Confusion
- Irritability
- Anxiety or panic attacks
- Seasonal allergies
- Runny nose and congestion
- Headaches and migraines (see sidebar, page 17)
- Acid reflux or other digestive issues (like nausea and vomiting)
- Abnormal menstrual cycle
- Loss of consciousness (rare)

SYMPTOMS OF
HISTAMINE INTOLERANCE

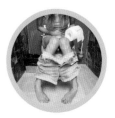

DIARRHEA

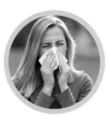

**HEADACHES/
MIGRAINES**

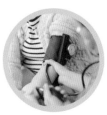

**CONGESTION/
RUNNY NOSE**

**LOW BLOOD
PRESSURE**

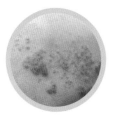

HIVES

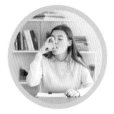

ASTHMA ATTACKS

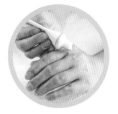

**ECZEMA/
PSORIASIS**

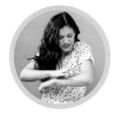

**CRAWLING SENSATIONS
ON SKIN OR SCALP**

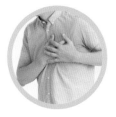

HYPERTENSION

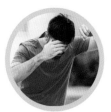

VERTIGO

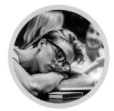

FATIGUE

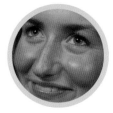

FLUSHING

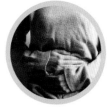

**ABNORMAL
MENSTRUAL CYCLE**

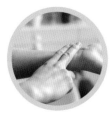

TACHYCARDIA

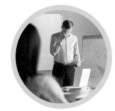

ANXIETY

Other reactions to histamine intolerance include the following:

- Sleep disturbances. Researchers have found that mast cells play a major role in running our internal clock. The cells actually have their own internal clock, which is controlled by a specific set of genes as well as by external factors, such as stress and diet. Combine this mechanism with the fact that histamine from mast cells in the brain can promote wakefulness and changes in behavioral states and you have a recipe for sleep disturbances and insomnia, creating a vicious cycle.
- Anxiety. Histamine acts as a neurotransmitter in the brain, which is why it can cause a chain reaction that can bring on anxiety, depression and other psychiatric conditions. A hypothalamic-pituitary-adrenal (HPA) axis imbalance can also increase the number of mast cells in the brain, bringing on anxiety-like behavior.

WHY VERTIGO AND MIGRAINES ARE SYMPTOMS OF HISTAMINE INTOLERANCE

Vertigo or dizziness can be caused by histamine release in the body, which is why some people with histamine intolerance frequently feel dizzy. It is also why many people who suffer from allergies often feel as if their ears are clogged, leading to that dizzy, unbalanced feeling. Allergies affect the Eustachian tubes in your ears, which help regulate your balance. When these tubes become filled with mucus due to histamine release or your body responding to an allergen, it can throw your balance off.

Migraine headaches can be caused by histamine intolerance and a buildup of nitrate oxide. Endothelial monoxide is released by histamine. Headaches can also be triggered by consuming histamine-rich foods. Many migraine sufferers also have reduced DAO activity.

HISTAMINE INTOLERANCE QUIZ

Take this quiz to help you determine whether you may be suffering from histamine intolerance.

1. Do you ever get fatigued after eating certain foods other than high-sugar foods?

2. Does your nose ever run while you are eating certain foods?

3. Do you suffer from vertigo or dizziness?

4. Do you ever feel tightening in your throat after eating (or even randomly)?

5. Do you have low blood pressure?

6. Do you suffer from migraine headaches?

7. Do you have skin issues like eczema, dermatitis or psoriasis?

8. Do you experience anxiety or panic attacks?

9. Do you experience any unwanted symptoms after eating fermented foods?

10. Do you experience any unwanted symptoms after eating leftover foods?

11. Does your face get red easily and stay that way during or after a workout?

If you answered yes to 0–1 of these questions, you may not be suffering from histamine intolerance.

If you answered yes to 2–5 of these questions, you most likely are suffering from histamine intolerance.

If you answered yes to more than 5 of these questions, you may be suffering from severe histamine intolerance.

WHY YOU MAY NOT HAVE BEEN TESTED FOR HISTAMINE INTOLERANCE

As you can see, histamine intolerance symptoms can range from minor to severe, and they can affect the entire body. Histamine travels through the bloodstream, so it can go everywhere that is nourished by your blood.

Histamine's widespread presence is also why diagnosing an intolerance can be a challenge. It can be hard to pinpoint the symptoms and link them back to having too much histamine in the body. Also, symptoms usually occur only once histamine hits a certain threshold, further complicating a diagnosis. You may not suffer from immediate symptoms even after consuming a histamine-rich food.

Many people also associate histamine intolerance with a food allergy because the symptoms can be similar. However, the difference between histamine intolerance and a true allergic reaction is that an intolerance to too much histamine is not an immediate hypersensitivity response, a true allergic reaction is. IgE are antibodies produced by the immune system—when you consume a food you are allergic to, your body produces IgE antibodies. These antibodies then travel to cells and cause an allergic reaction. However, with histamine intolerance, the reaction is not mediated by IgE in the same way that an allergic reaction is, and because symptoms may not be immediate, it may be difficult to determine which foods trigger a reaction.

Often, it can be difficult trying to determine which foods you react poorly to if you are not keeping a detailed food journal. You may consume a histamine-rich meal for dinner but not experience symptoms until the next morning. Without a food journal, it could be very easy to dismiss the morning symptoms and not link it to the foods you ate the night before. This is why I always recommend keeping a detailed food journal when dealing with histamine intolerance, but more on that later.

DOWNLOAD FOOD JOURNAL

http://bit.ly/HITjournal

Because of the difficulty of diagnosing histamine intolerance, it may be necessary to work with a skilled practitioner who is able to help determine whether this is, in fact, your issue. Still, there are problems with the tests available. Many of them are unreliable, and others are unable to properly detect the level of histamine present in your body at any one time.

The most reliable test I have found aims to determine how the intestinal barrier is holding up. Because leaky gut (intestinal permeability) can be a big cause of histamine intolerance, this test can be a great way to uncover the source of your issues. It looks for the following:

- Level of histamine
- Level of DAO (the enzyme that breaks down histamine)
- The DAO-to-histamine ratio (which helps detect imbalances between DAO and histamine)
- Level of lipopolysaccharide (which is another marker for leaky gut because it is produced from bacterial cell walls and initiates an inflammatory response in the body)
- Zonulin (a compound responsible for opening up the tiny holes, or tight junctions, in the intestinal barrier, leading to leaky gut)

I think the easiest and most cost-effective way to determine histamine intolerance is to test how you react to fermented foods. Most people who have histamine intolerance cannot tolerate them and will note this by expressing one or more of the symptoms listed on page 15.

You can also follow a low-histamine diet like the plan I offer in this book to see how you feel. If your symptoms subside, there's a good chance you suffer from histamine intolerance and would benefit from some form of the diet long term. Whether you have to follow a low-histamine diet long term is largely determined by how well you can follow the other lifestyle changes I am going to talk about in this book.

It's also useful to assess risk factors when determining whether you might have histamine intolerance.

RISK FACTORS FOR HISTAMINE INTOLERANCE

You may be more likely than other people to have histamine intolerance for a range of reasons. If you are suffering from chronic stress, sleep disturbances, anxiety, thyroid dysfunction or other conditions, you could be at higher risk for developing histamine intolerance.

STRESS AND HPA-AXIS DYSFUNCTION

High stress levels can have a huge impact on histamine production in the body, so stress can also affect which foods you are able to consume safely (that is, without a reaction).

Stress is a risk factor that deserves a lot of attention. It increases inflammation, putting a heavy burden on the body. This is why, in addition to reducing high-histamine foods, you will see that I also have you eliminate inflammatory foods to help reduce the inflammation load. We will go into a lot more detail about inflammatory foods soon.

The HPA axis is responsible for responding during periods of stress. In the event of stress, the adrenal glands kick in to high gear and can put the body in a fight-or-flight mode as a protective mechanism when there is a real threat. The problem is that many people go into fight-or-flight mode with a perceived threat rather than an actual threat. The adrenals respond to both kinds of threats equally. When under chronic stress, the body no longer knows how to differentiate between real and perceived threats and things like heart rate and blood pressure become perpetually elevated.

Constant stress overtaxes your adrenal glands, leading you to feel jittery or experience insomnia. The HPA axis can become so exhausted from the incessant stress that it decreases activity, which many people experience as adrenal fatigue. Those with HPA-axis dysfunction may be overburdened with histamine and not have the ability to break it down properly. The inability to break down histamine can make symptoms of HPA-axis dysfunction worse, and any type of HPA-axis dysfunction can lead to other health issues.

Stress also causes the mast cells to degranulate (break open) and release histamine and other inflammatory chemicals into the body. In response, the adrenals release more and more cortisol, an anti-inflammatory agent, essentially making the adrenal glands work overtime.

THE STRESS-HISTAMINE
CONNECTION

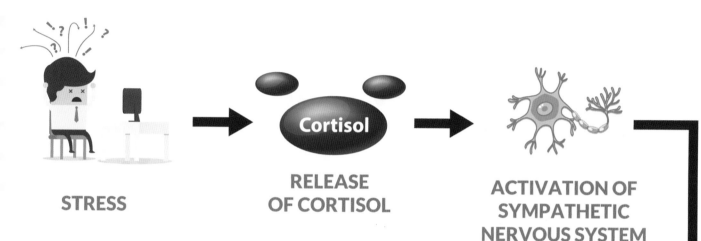

STRESS → **RELEASE OF CORTISOL** → **ACTIVATION OF SYMPATHETIC NERVOUS SYSTEM**

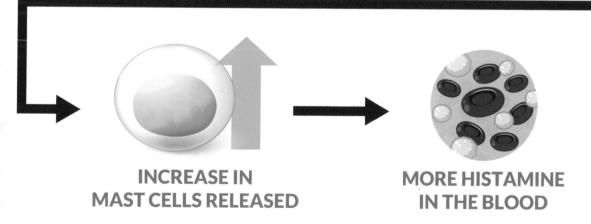

INCREASE IN MAST CELLS RELEASED → **MORE HISTAMINE IN THE BLOOD**

GENETIC POLYMORPHISM

Having a genetic polymorphism can put you at an increased risk for developing histamine intolerance. You can learn more about this specific gene mutation that puts you at a greater risk in Chapter 2 (page 45).

CERTAIN MEDICATIONS

Certain medications, including antacids, antibiotics and antihistamines, can inhibit DAO enzyme activity and thereby increase histamine production. You can find a full list of medications that inhibit DAO in Chapter 2 (page 47).

HORMONAL IMBALANCES

Having a hormone imbalance, particularly estrogen dominance, can lead to histamine intolerance. Estrogen dominance is a common hormonal imbalance in industrialized countries and plays a role in many conditions, including premenstrual syndrome (PMS), polycystic ovary syndrome (PCOS), uterine fibroids, breast cancer and cystic breast disease in women. In men, it can cause the growth of male breasts and larger hips, reduce testosterone and lead to emotional disturbances. The symptoms of estrogen dominance also include the following:

- Decreased sex drive
- Sluggish metabolism
- Fatigue
- Insomnia
- Brain fog
- Breast swelling and tenderness
- Irregular or abnormal menstrual periods
- Irritability and depression
- Weight gain
- Headaches

Factors that contribute to estrogen dominance include chronic stress, obesity, poor diet or digestive function, birth control pills, lack of exercise and ingestion of environmental estrogens. These environmental estrogens can come from simple items we use every day, including nail polishes, plastics, perfumes, new carpets, fabric softeners and many different types of cosmetics. This is why I recommend choosing natural options where possible and making your own beauty and household products.

It has been found that estrogen triggers histamine release and that histamine causes an increase in estrogen. The two reinforce each other. Essentially, if you have too much estrogen, your body is likely to be releasing too much histamine.

However, that's not the only link between estrogen dominance and histamine intolerance. Estrogen is thought to affect the immune system—specifically mast cells, which we know release histamine when the immune system is activated. It has been found that estrogen in the form of estradiol can activate mast cells. Estrogen can also interfere with how DAO and monoamine oxidase (MAO, another enzyme that breaks down histamine) work, which are important for breaking down histamine.

Knowing this information, it makes sense why many women suffer from symptoms related to histamine intolerance right before ovulation.

HISTAMINE-THYROID

CONNECTION

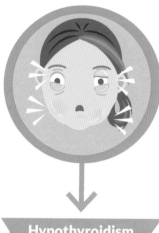

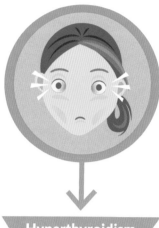

Hypothyroidism

Hyperthyroidism

Increase in Mast Cell Production

Increase in Histamine Receptors

Increase in Histamine Production

Plus ↓ DAO and/or DAO Mutation

Increased Response to Histamine in the Body

Histamine Intolerance

Development of Autoimmune Thyroid Disorders

THYROID DYSFUNCTION

Many people don't know that thyroid dysfunction can play a role in histamine intolerance and vice versa. In hypothyroidism, low levels of the thyroid hormone can increase mast cell activity, which increases the amount of histamine in the body. With hyperthyroidism, too much thyroid hormone can increase the number of histamine receptors in the body, which can cause an increased response to histamine. Add a decrease in the DAO enzyme to the mix and you can have yourself a case of histamine intolerance. It has also been found that high levels of histamine in the body can lead to autoimmune conditions like Hashimoto's disease. Furthermore, the same things that can cause histamine intolerance—like SIBO, leaky gut and more—can trigger thyroid dysfunction in the body as well.

ENVIRONMENTAL ALLERGEN EXPOSURE

Frequent exposure to things like pollen, mold and dust mites can put you at risk for histamine intolerance. It may be difficult to determine when these substances are in your environment, but the symptoms that you experience may be very obvious.

LIFESTYLE FACTORS

Burning yourself out with too much exercise (specifically aerobic exercise) can increase histamine levels in the body, a problem for those suffering from histamine intolerance. This doesn't mean you should completely avoid exercise, but doing lower-impact workouts or doing more weight training and yoga instead of high-intensity aerobic exercise may be a better choice.

Another lifestyle factor that could contribute to histamine intolerance is consuming too much alcohol. Alcohol is high in histamine and a histamine liberator (releasing the histamine in our body), so it should be avoided or limited.

Two

THE EIGHT MOST COMMON CAUSES **OF HISTAMINE** INTOLERANCE

Some of the underlying factors we discuss in this section may cause histamine intolerance as they decrease DAO function, while others directly affect how much histamine is released in the body. Some people may be affected by one underlying cause on this list, while others may be affected by a handful of them.

WORKING WITH A PROFESSIONAL VERSUS TREATING YOURSELF AT HOME

When dealing with histamine intolerance, if you can get to the root of the issue and eliminate the foods that are triggering your symptoms, you should be able to manage this condition very well. I have created an online program at DrBeckyCampbell.com to help you not only uncover what your triggers are but also determine the tests you need and specific treatment protocols based on your personal test results. There are cases in which someone may need to work with a skilled practitioner, but my goal is to help you manage this the best you can on your own.

CAUSE 1
MAST CELL ACTIVATION SYNDROME

I believe that Mast Cell Activation Syndrome (MCAS) is the primary cause of histamine intolerance, but it may not be the cause for everyone. Mast cells are white blood cells that are present in tissues throughout the body. Large numbers of mast cells can be found in the skin, respiratory tract, digestive tract, urinary tract, reproductive organs and surrounding nerves. They can also be found in blood and in the body as a result of things like infections and diseases. Mast cells begin repairing tissues once the threat is gone.

Mast cells are also involved in allergic reactions. They store inflammatory mediators inside granules that also include histamine. During an allergic reaction, or in the case of infection or disease, mast cells are activated and the contents of their granules are released into the surrounding tissues. This is what triggers symptoms linked to inflammation as well as an allergic response.

MOST COMMON CAUSES OF

HISTAMINE INTOLERANCE

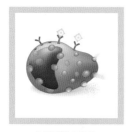

**MAST CELL
ACTIVATION SYNDROME**

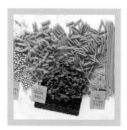

GLUTEN INTOLERANCE

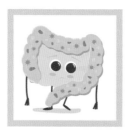

LEAKY GUT

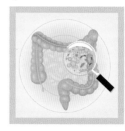

GUT INFECTIONS

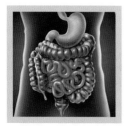

**INFLAMMATORY
DIGESTIVE DISEASES**

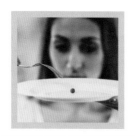

NUTRIENT DEFICIENCIES

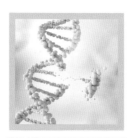

GENETIC MUTATIONS

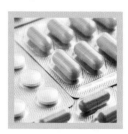

CERTAIN MEDICATIONS

The difference between the two can be thought of in this way: histamine intolerance involves adding more histamine to the body (for instance, with certain foods), causing a buildup in the body that the body has trouble breaking down. This is different to how MCAS works. With MCAS, mast cells are triggered and spill chemicals into your body, one of which is histamine, causing a wide range of symptoms.

Your body can send any of more than 200 signals to mast cells, and many of the 25 to 50 known mast cell triggers can come from your environment. Some of them include the following:

- Mold
- Allergens
- Viruses
- Chemicals and toxins
- Heavy metals

While not all people with histamine intolerance have MCAS, if you do have both conditions, your body will not be able to properly break down that extra histamine, which will lead to a buildup quite quickly.

- Fatigue
- Weakness
- Dizziness

Note the similarity of the preceding symptoms to the symptoms of histamine intolerance. The effects of the two can be very similar due to the increased amount of histamine in the body that both conditions involve.

CONDITIONS ASSOCIATED WITH MCAS

MCAS is related to a number of different conditions, including the following:

- Allergies and asthma
- Eczema
- Ehlers-Danlos syndrome (EDS)
- Chronic fatigue syndrome
- Chronic inflammatory response syndrome
- Fibromyalgia
- Infertility (mast cells in the endometrium may contribute to endometriosis)
- Interstitial cystitis
- Celiac disease
- Eosinophilic esophagitis
- Food allergies and intolerances
- Gastroesophageal reflux
- Irritable bowel syndrome
- Migraine headaches
- Autism
- Mood disorders (insomnia, anxiety, depression)
- Postural orthostatic tachycardia syndrome
- Multiple chemical sensitivities
- Autoimmune diseases (Hashimoto's thyroiditis, systemic lupus, multiple sclerosis, bullous pemphigoid, rheumatoid arthritis and others)

THE UNDERLYING CAUSES OF MCAS

Some of the underlying causes of MCAS include a preexisting genetic disposition, gut microbiome dysbiosis, infections, stress and toxins.

Those with Ehlers-Danlos syndrome (EDS), a genetic disorder that causes joint hypermobility and changes in the immune system, are predisposed to MCAS. In one study, 66 percent of individuals with EDS had symptoms consistent with MCAS.

Infections like Lyme disease can also contribute to changes in the body and, in my opinion, the development of MCAS, and I have heard other practitioners say the same. People with MCAS may also frequently suffer from upper respiratory infections, high blood pressure and fibromyalgia.

Toxins like heavy metals, mold and other biotoxins can cause damage to the liver, affecting your body's ability to detoxify itself and becoming an underlying cause of MCAS. Stress can also play a key role, especially when it causes the body's hormonal system to get out of balance.

MASTOCYTOSIS

Mastocytosis is also worth mentioning here, as it shares some symptoms with MCAS, though it is a rare disorder that is usually caused by a genetic mutation. There are two types: cutaneous and systemic. Cutaneous mastocytosis occurs when mast cells accumulate in the skin; systemic mastocytosis occurs when mast cells accumulate in the internal organs like the liver, spleen, small intestine or bone marrow.

Cutaneous mastocytosis symptoms include the following:

- Flushing
- Redness
- Swelling

Systemic mastocytosis symptoms may include the following:

- Itching, hives and/or flushing of the skin
- Gastrointestinal symptoms like abdominal pain, diarrhea, nausea and vomiting
- Anemia and bleeding disorders
- Enlargement of the liver, spleen or lymph nodes

If you have mastocytosis, the recommendations in this book may also help you feel your best and minimize symptoms.

TESTING FOR MCAS

While it may be difficult to test for histamine intolerance, there are tests available for MCAS, including these:

- Serum tryptase (most famous mast cell mediator)
- Serum chromogranin A
- Plasma histamine
- Plasma PGD2 (chilled)
- Plasma heparin (chilled)
- Urine for PGD2 (chilled)
- PGF2a
- N-methylhistamine
- Biopsy (one of the best ways to diagnose MCAS)

However, testing is still not 100 percent accurate as I'm writing this. So it is a good idea to take advantage of the recommendations I make in this book no matter what laboratory test results come back for you. If you do have MCAS, more drastic measures may have to be taken and you may need to work with an MCAS specialist. I have listed a few of these specialists on page 179.

GETTING WELL

While MCAS can be more difficult to heal on your own, there are many things you can do to start feeling better right away. Following the plan laid out for histamine intolerance in this book could completely eliminate all symptoms.

CAUSE 2
GLUTEN INTOLERANCE

Gluten intolerance is on the rise, and more people are keeping this inflammatory substance out of their diet to the benefit of their health. Gluten can be found in the following grains:

- Wheat
- Rye
- Barley
- Malt
- Durum
- Semolina
- Farina
- Farro
- Graham
- Kamut

Common sources of gluten are pasta, bread, baked goods, crackers, croutons, flour-based products, cereal, brewer's yeast, beer and certain sauces and dressings. Classic gluten intolerance symptoms include digestive upset, skin issues, headaches and brain fog.

WHY GLUTEN IS USUALLY A PROBLEM

Gluten can be problematic for more than one reason. Apart from the fact that it is an inflammatory substance, it is especially harmful for those suffering from a thyroid condition, as the body can mistake gluten for healthy thyroid tissue and vice versa. When the body cannot differentiate between gluten and the thyroid, the body may mount an attack on both, causing thyroid damage. Gluten can also increase the release of zonulin, which opens the tight junctions in the gut. This can cause leaky gut syndrome.

WHY YOUR DOCTOR MAY NOT HAVE TESTED YOU FOR GLUTEN INTOLERANCE

If you suspect you may be dealing with gluten intolerance, you might be interested in testing. The problem with testing for gluten intolerance is that most doctors—especially in the world of conventional medicine—will only test for two markers and will focus on ruling out celiac disease as opposed to looking for gluten intolerance.

Your doctor may run a transglutaminase 2 autoantibody test. If it is positive, your doctor may then perform a small-intestine biopsy. However, it is very important to get the right testing done if you suspect that you may be dealing with gluten intolerance and not true celiac disease, because you can have one without the other.

Why is it that many conventional-medicine doctors won't test for gluten sensitivity? While it is accepted that celiac disease is a condition, nonceliac gluten sensitivity is simply not as widely accepted among those working in the conventional-medicine field. Celiac disease is an autoimmune condition in which the immune system will respond to the ingestion of gluten as well as related proteins while also harming the gut tissue. Nonceliac gluten sensitivity (a.k.a. nonceliac wheat sensitivity), on the other hand, involves the development of symptoms like fatigue and brain fog after the consumption of gluten, without any of the classic markers of celiac disease.

Unless you are seeing an experienced functional-medicine practitioner, you may find it very difficult to get a diagnosis. However, this doesn't mean that nonceliac gluten sensitivity doesn't exist. In fact, in my experience, people who suffer from gluten sensitivity usually feel much better when they cut gluten out of their diet, and the aforementioned symptoms begin to fade away.

TESTING FOR GLUTEN INTOLERANCE

I mainly run the Cyrex Laboratories' Array 3 test on my patients to test for nonceliac gluten sensitivity. I use this test because it looks at the antibody production against different wheat proteins, the gliadin-transglutaminase complex, as well as three important enzymes that all help diagnose wheat or gluten sensitivity. However, the test isn't always necessary, because eliminating gluten is almost always beneficial. I always recommend that my patients eliminate gluten so they can experience the benefits that elimination can bring.

GETTING WELL

Start by removing gluten from your diet completely. See the list on page 57.

CAUSE 3
LEAKY GUT

Leaky gut is a condition in which the barrier of the intestines, which runs from the mouth to the anus, becomes "leaky." Every healthy individual actually has small holes in their intestines, but in people with leaky gut, these holes become large and can cause severe symptoms. The large holes allow undigested foods, bacteria and other toxins to leak into the bloodstream. When these foreign substances gain access in this way, they can trigger an autoimmune reaction in the body and create inflammation, skin issues, fatigue, digestive complaints, food allergies and histamine intolerance. Having a leaky gut can also make it very difficult for your body to absorb certain key nutrients, leading to vitamin and mineral deficiencies. Leaky gut is another underlying cause of low DAO, the enzyme that breaks down histamine, as any type of inflammation in the body can impede DAO function.

The Cyrex Laboratories' Array 2 test is different. It looks at specific antibodies to proteins and bacterial endotoxins, which are both very important pieces to the leaky gut puzzle. It allows a more thorough diagnosis, because having these proteins or toxins transfer from the gut into the bloodstream can trigger an inflammatory reaction and possibly an autoimmune disease.

However, having testing done may not be totally necessary, especially if it is something you don't want to invest money in. You may not need a test to tell you definitively, because the symptoms of leaky gut can help diagnose the condition. Changing your diet and starting a healing protocol may be beneficial for more than one area of your life, whether you have leaky gut or not.

GETTING WELL

There are several things you can do to support leaky gut.

START AN ELIMINATION DIET. Starting an elimination diet is a great way to help support leaky gut. I recommend eliminating gluten, grains, sugar, dairy and soy, as all of these are inflammatory and many people react to these foods. Food additives should also be removed from the diet, as well as pesticides, hormones, antibiotics and steroids found in conventional animal products.

I recommend removing all of these foods from your diet for at least 60 days; then, if you choose to reintroduce them, try reintroducing just one food from each food group at a time and not introduce anything else for 3 days. However, I recommend keeping all gluten, soy, grains and refined sugar out of your diet long term and following a Paleo-style, low-histamine diet generally. Following a Paleo diet will help further reduce inflammation and support gut health.

permeability to large molecules that would cause inflammation. It is great for anyone who has been suffering from leaky gut symptoms—such as chronic fatigue, brain fog or food sensitivities—or any type of autoimmune disease.

There's another test called the lactulose-mannitol test that was used quite often in the case of suspected leaky gut, but it is not something I use in my practice because there are quite a few problems with this test. For one, lactulose and mannitol are small molecules, so it's possible that the test would not produce any type of immune reaction. Not only that, but the transfer of lactulose or mannitol through the gut barrier is not necessarily indicative of leaky gut, so a positive result may not be enough to indicate a definitive leaky gut diagnosis.

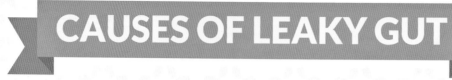

CAUSES OF LEAKY GUT

INFLAMMATORY FOODS:

| Sugar | Alcohol | Dairy | Grain | Gluten |

MEDICATIONS:

| NSAIDS | Steroids | Antibiotics | Birth Control | Antacids |

GUT INFECTIONS:

 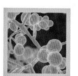

Bacterial Dysbiosis — Yeast Infections — Intestinal Parasites — Small Intestinal Bacteria Overgrowth (SIBO)

ENVIRONMENTAL TOXINS:

Mercury (heavy metal toxicity) — Plastics — BPAs

CHRONIC STRESS:

Continual stress will decrease the effectiveness of your immune system, making it more difficult for your body to fight bacteria and viruses, leading to more systemic inflammation, including the gut lining.

dida can all make these conditions worse. But by getting the right testing, you can uncover potential infections and then treat them at their source. I talk more specifically about SIBO, parasites and candida (as well as options for testing) later in this chapter.

ELIMINATE NSAID AND ALCOHOL USE. NSAIDs like aspirin and ibuprofen can be problematic for those dealing with leaky gut syndrome. NSAIDs can block the body's ability to produce prostaglandins, the substances needed to help rebuild the intestinal lining. Taking NSAIDs for even just a two-week period can cause a problem. If you take NSAIDs regularly, do what you can to reduce the amount you take as much as possible, especially if you have the symptoms of leaky gut.

Alcohol can also be an issue. Alcohol is very hard on the gut lining and may further damage the intestinal membrane. I recommend steering clear of alcohol, or at least significantly cutting back, when dealing with leaky gut.

in another.

DOWNLOAD FOOD JOURNAL

http://bit.ly/HITjournal

The same goes for leaky gut. When dealing with this condition, you may be suffering from multiple food sensitivities that may not be causing symptoms right away. By tracking your food intake, you will be able to better pinpoint which foods you should avoid and which foods are safe for you to enjoy.

UNCOVER GUT INFECTIONS. Many people with leaky gut or histamine intolerance also have hidden gut infections. Things like SIBO, parasites and can-

ADD MORE WHOLE FOODS TO YOUR DIET. Whether you are dealing with leaky gut or not, adding more whole foods to your diet can be extremely beneficial. I strongly encourage removing as many processed and artificial foods from your diet as you can as well as maintaining a whole-foods, low-histamine diet to improve your health quickly. Whole foods will help repair the gut lining, whereas processed foods can make leaky gut damage worse. Whole foods like fruits, vegetables, healthy fats and clean proteins are full of nutrition your body needs to thrive and function at its best.

In order for your body and gut to heal, you will need to fuel your body properly. Keep reading to learn about specific foods tailored to a low-histamine plan.

REDUCE STRESS. Have you ever noticed that when you are stressed, stomach issues start popping up? For some, this takes the form of nausea and diarrhea or even stomach pain and acid reflux. When you are constantly stressed, your body is likely in a state of fight-or-flight as opposed to where you really want your nervous system to be: in rest-and-digest mode to support gut healing and overall health.

The only way to help calm your nervous system is to reduce stress as much as possible and to dedicate some time each day to doing so. Try doing yoga, meditation, reading or even brisk walking to help calm your mind and check out from the stressors in your life. Focusing on reducing stress for even just fifteen minutes each day can help.

SUPPLEMENTATION

A great way to support gut healing is to supplement appropriately. I recommend a supplement with the following ingredients to help support the gut lining.

L-Glutamine

L-glutamine is an amino acid found in the body that helps support digestive and immune health. It can help heal the cells in the small intestine, which is important for those dealing with a leaky gut.

Deglycyrrhizinated Licorice

Deglycyrrhizinated licorice (DGL) is an adaptogenic herb that is commonly used to support healthy mucosal lining of both the gut and the duodenum. Keep in mind that licorice candy contains glycyrrhizin, which can cause high blood pressure, so it is best to stick with DGL in herb form.

Aloe Vera Gel Extract

Aloe vera is commonly recognized as a sunburn remedy, but it can actually be very helpful for supporting leaky gut too. Aloe vera has anti-inflammatory properties and helps maintain the acid-alkaline balance in the gut.

Zinc Carnosine

Zinc carnosine is an essential trace element, and deficiency is common. It has been shown to help support a healthy gut lining and is commonly known for its wound-healing properties, making it great for mucosal healing too.

ULTIMATE GUT SUPPORT

Conveniently, all of these supplements (and others) can be found in my Ultimate Gut Support supplement. The lining of the gut must have proper permeability so that it can prevent toxins, microbes and allergens from getting into the bloodstream and absorb nutrients. Learn more about this supplement on page 175.

- Nausea
- Frequent burping
- Bloating
- Unexplained weight loss
- Loss of appetite
- Abdominal pain that's worse when your stomach is empty
- An aching or burning sensation in your abdomen

You can be exposed to the bacteria via utensils, food, water and saliva from an infected person. Many people live with *H. pylori* yet experience no symptoms, or they experience reflux and heartburn but are never tested for this bacterium, so its presence goes undetected.

H. PYLORI AND HISTAMINE

Although research into the connection between *H. pylori* and histamine is in its initial stages, we do know that *H. pylori* causes more histamine to be produced by mast cells in the gut lining. We also know that *H. pylori* makes the gut lining more permeable, and the undigested food particles allowed through can stimulate allergic reactions. The bacteria literally drill tiny holes in your gut, exposing you to all the dangers of leaky gut syndrome.

An *H. pylori* infection has also been linked to lower stomach acid levels, fatigue, parasites, mineral deficiencies, autoimmune disorders, liver problems and a host of other issues. It tends to get worse over time if not treated, which means your histamine intolerance symptoms are also likely to increase over time if the *H. pylori* infection isn't addressed.

TESTING FOR H. PYLORI

Doing the proper testing to find out if you have *H. pylori* is important. Most labs can do a test for *H. pylori.* Your doctor will have you take a breath test, stool test or blood test.

SUPPLEMENTATION

Mastic gum, methylmethionine sulfonium (vitamin U) and DGL have been used successfully to treat *H. pylori*. Other beneficial supplements include black seed (Nigella sativa), broccoli sprouts, garlic, propolis and goldenseal.

GETTING WELL

Reducing stress is beneficial when you have *H. pylori*, as stress only makes your symptoms worse and upsets your natural immune response.

SIBO

SIBO is a condition in which the mechanism that usually prevents the buildup of bacteria in the small intestine fails to work, leading to overgrowth. Although you are supposed to have a small amount of bacteria in your small intestine, the majority should be in your colon. Some people with SIBO have too much hydrochloric acid (HCL), which is produced in the body to help with digestion; but most SIBO sufferers actually have too little, a condition called hypochlorhydria. Without enough stomach acid, foods simply aren't broken down properly. And with improper digestion, undigested foods can ferment, leading to further discomfort and potential bacteria buildup in the small intestine. Thus, some of the common symptoms of SIBO include the following:

- Abdominal pain
- Bloating
- Diarrhea or constipation (diarrhea is much more common)
- Irritable bowel syndrome or irritable bowel disease
- Weight loss
- Fatigue
- Malnutrition
- Skin issues (acne, eczema, rashes, rosacea)
- Asthma
- Depression
- Food sensitivities

SIBO AND HISTAMINE

How is SIBO connected with histamine intolerance? As we have already talked about, certain types of gut bacteria have the ability to produce histamine. When a person is dealing with SIBO, the gut microbes in their digestive system may produce large amounts of histamine. When this happens, the DAO enzyme may not be able to get rid of all the histamine that's released, leading to gut dysfunction. The histamine can also circulate throughout the bloodstream and get into different areas in the body, causing symptoms like headache, eczema, irritability, difficult breathing or asthma.

ROOT CAUSES OF SIBO

Certain medications—such as immunosuppressant drugs and proton pump inhibitors like omeprazole—can cause SIBO. It can also be caused by abdominal surgery, celiac disease, diabetes, diverticulosis and pancreatitis. Aging can be another contributing factor simply because our digestive system starts to slow down. In addition, low HCL levels can be an underlying cause of SIBO.

TESTING FOR SIBO

If you suspect you may be dealing with SIBO, the tests I recommend include the lactulose breath test from NUNM SIBO Lab or BioHealth Laboratory and a blood test available through Cyrex Laboratories. You can order these tests in my online program.

Testing for SIBO can be tricky because the testing is not always reliable. The lactulose breath test is a noninvasive test in which the patient consumes lactulose. Lactulose is poorly absorbed from our GI tract because we do not have the enzymes necessary to break it down. This means the lactulose will travel to the end of the small intestine unchanged, which will help diagnose any type of bacterial overgrowth present in the distal part of the small intestine.

Some doctors use the glucose breath test, but this test has its disadvantages. Because glucose is digestible, it may be digested before it even reaches the distal end of the small intestine, making it more difficult to detect bacterial overgrowth.

move gluten, grains, sugar and dairy from your et. Take digestive enzymes with betaine HCL (see e previous section). Review all of the medications u are taking to see whether there is a link between e of them and a possible underlying trigger of BO.

ANDIDA AND SMALL INTESTINE UNGAL OVERGROWTH

andida is another underlying cause of histamine tolerance that is all too common. Candida is a ungus that helps with nutrient absorption as well as digestion, but when it is present in excess amounts, t can break down the walls of the intestinal lining and get into the bloodstream. This causes the release of by-product toxins and can lead to leaky gut. Some of the classic symptoms of candida overgrowth include the following:

- Craving sweet foods
- Bad breath
- White coating on the tongue (also known as oral thrush)
- Hormone imbalances
- Chronic fatigue
- Weakened immune system
- Frequent gas and bloating
- Brain fog
- Joint pain
- Decreased sex drive
- Frequent urinary tract infections

Keep in mind that the preceding symptoms can be related to a lot of different things, such as parasites (page 40). This is why it is important not to treat the condition solely based on symptoms and why testing is key.

- Undecylenic acid
- Grapefruit seed extract
- Berberine
- Monolaurin
- Partially hydrogenated guar gum
- Atrantil (I usually recommend this supplement during the second round of treatment if SIBO is still present, after using other supplement options for at least 60 days.)

Do not start taking all of these supplements just because you suspect you have SIBO. Many gut issues can mimic one another, so testing is extremely important to make the proper diagnosis. There are also many combination supplements, and the right practitioner or my online program can help you determine the proper protocol for you.

Small intestine fungal overgrowth (SIFO) is another type of fungal overgrowth that Chris Kresser, a leading expert in functional medicine, and a few other practitioners are starting to talk about. This condition is similar to SIBO, but the overgrowth is fungal instead of bacterial. Some patients who have unexplained gastrointestinal issues and who do not get better from treatment may be suffering from SIFO. This condition is often missed and is commonly misdiagnosed as SIBO.

ROOT CAUSES OF CANDIDA

There are a couple potential root causes of candida overgrowth. Taking antibiotics, especially frequently and for long periods of time, is one of the main ones. Antibiotics kill the bad bacteria as well as the good bacteria in your digestive system. This becomes a problem because one of the roles of the good bacteria in your gut is to keep candida growth under control.

Taking birth control pills is another key risk factor. Some women experience more frequent yeast infections when taking birth control pills. Another class of medications we need to watch out for are oral corticosteroids. Things like inhalers can lead to an oral candida overgrowth if you don't follow the proper precaution of swishing your mouth with water after each use.

Other candida risk factors include having diabetes, a weakened immune system or an autoimmune disease.

CANDIDA AND HISTAMINE

Now that we know a little bit more about candida, let's talk about the link between candida overgrowth and histamine intolerance. Candida is not only a problem in and of itself but it is also an issue for those dealing with a histamine intolerance because it can make the intolerance worse. Candida may be able to trigger histamine release because, as with any infection, the immune system responds and histamine is released. Studies have found that a candida infection can trigger mast cells to release mediators while working to kill off the infection. The problem is that histamine lives in mast cells, so when tons of mast cells respond to an infection like candida overgrowth, lots of histamine may be released. As you can see, this would be a problem for someone with histamine intolerance. A candida infection can also reduce DAO enzymes, decreasing your ability to properly break down histamine.

TESTING FOR CANDIDA

If you suffer from candida overgrowth, it is vital to get the infection under control as a way to help reduce the amount of histamine in your body. If you suspect you have candida, I personally recommend specialty stool tests, which can detect fungal overgrowth in the stool. Blood tests can check for antibodies against candida. However, one of the drawbacks of a blood test is that you won't know whether there is a current infection or whether the antibodies are from a past candida infection. Finally, urine testing can be helpful because d-arabinitol, an organic acid marker found in urine, can help detect fungal overgrowth.

Despite these options, there is no perfect test. Each test has its own downsides, but the stool and urine tests in particular can be helpful with diagnosing candida.

THE IMPORTANCE OF DIET WHEN TREATING CANDIDA

If you are suffering from candida, there are some steps you can take to help get it under control. The first place to start is diet. I will talk in much more detail about the importance of a low-histamine diet and how to start one in the coming chapters, but in the case of candida, it is vital to eliminate sugar, alcohol and refined carbohydrates. These all contribute to candida overgrowth and must be removed from your diet to get the infection under control. Replace these foods with whole, nourishing, low-histamine and anti-inflammatory foods to combat candida infection.

It is also important to mention that you do not need to eliminate all carbs to get rid of candida. I use a low-carb diet approach in my practice instead of a no-carb (candida) diet.

GETTING WELL

If you are suffering from candida overgrowth, know that there are natural ways to assist the healing process, and the sooner you get the infection under control, the better you will feel. By supplementing appropriately, getting the proper testing and making the necessary dietary changes, you can take the steps needed to reduce candida as well as histamine in your body. Keep reading to learn about a specific low-histamine dietary plan that can be implemented that will also help with an underlying candida infection.

SUPPLEMENTATION

There are also some natural supplements you can take. Conventional-medicine doctors are likely to prescribe antifungal medications, but candida infections are often resistant to these antifungal drugs. Instead, I recommend the following powerful supplements to my patients with candida.

Coconut Oil

Coconut oil is one of the most popular options for fighting a candida infection. It is rich in caprylic and lauric acids, which act as natural antifungals. Certain extracts can also offer enhanced effects. Monolaurin and caprylic acid supplements, for example, allow you to get higher levels of lauric and caprylic acid than coconut oil alone.

Oregano and Thyme Oils

Oregano oil is commonly used to help support the immune system and fight off infection, which is why it is so beneficial for those with candida overgrowth. Thyme oil can also be beneficial, but please know that both oregano and thyme oil are very powerful, so it is best to work with a health-care practitioner before using them.

Biofilm Disruptors

Yeast can form a biofilm to live in, making it harder for your immune system or natural antimicrobials to get rid of the excess yeast. A biofilm-disrupting supplement may therefore be helpful. N-acetylcysteine and Biofilm Defense work well.

Keep in mind that I recommend working with a practitioner before starting any new supplement. There are a number of botanicals that work well to fight candida:

- Cat's claw
- Uva ursi
- Chinese skullcap
- Pau d'arco
- Coptis
- Berberine
- Oregon grape

PARASITES

Parasites are not something that many of us like to talk about. We fear them, and many people think they can only get them from traveling to a foreign country. However, the truth is that I see many patients who have parasites and don't even know they have them!

When people think about parasites, they often think of worms, but things like protozoa and yeast are also considered intestinal parasites. What all parasites have in common is that they steal nutrients and beneficial bacteria from the gut and rely on their hosts (us) to stay alive.

WORMS

Worms are parasites that can be acquired from food sources like unwashed fruits and vegetables and uncooked or undercooked meats. There are also different types of worms, including roundworms, tapeworms, pinworms and hookworms. The worms' eggs are ingested and then these eggs hatch inside the intestines. What's even worse is that you become sick from the worms when their fecal matter is absorbed through the intestines and enters the bloodstream.

Intestinal worms also eat the food you consume before your body gets a chance to absorb it, which can lead to malnourishment. In some cases, if gone untreated for long periods of time, parasitic worms can lead to organ damage if they wind up in the bloodstream or the liver. Unfortunately, worms are much more common than we may think and can be easily acquired from a variety of foods.

PROTOZOA

A protozoa parasitic infection comes from contaminated water. Contaminated water can cause giardia, which can cause severe digestive distress, including diarrhea, cramping and nausea. All of these symptoms combined can lead to dehydration.

SYMPTOMS OF PARASITES

Parasitic infections can cause a whole host of symptoms and issues. Some of the most common symptoms include these:

- Digestive health issues (diarrhea, constipation, nausea, gas, yeast infection)
- Chronic allergies
- Skin issues
- Anxiety, depression, confusion
- Fatigue
- Weight loss
- Appetite changes (both a loss of appetite or a feeling like you are not able to satisfy your hunger)
- Anemia
- Rectal itching
- Circles under the eyes
- Bad breath

Many of these symptoms are caused by the parasites stealing the nutrients you consume, leading to malnourishment. Other symptoms, such as digestive distress, may be directly caused by the infection itself. However, remember to look for symptoms and test, don't guess!

HOW DO WE GET PARASITES?

We talked about how worms are commonly acquired through ingesting infected foods, but there are other ways we can contract parasites. In my practice, the majority of my patients with parasites have cats. This is because transmitting a parasite is very easy and can be done by simply petting an infected pet. Contaminated water is also a source of parasites. Young children, because they may not wash their hands as frequently as older children and adults, tend to spread parasites through the skin by touching.

PARASITES AND HISTAMINE

Now that we know a bit more about parasites and how we get them, let's talk about how they are linked to histamine intolerance. Remember that mast cells release histamine as well as other inflammatory agents during an immune response? Well, mast cells release histamine to help fight off certain infections, including parasites. For those who are dealing with histamine intolerance, the excessive amount of histamine released by mast cells can lead to a whole host of symptoms because the histamine won't be broken down properly.

TESTING FOR PARASITES

I always use the GI-Map stool tests. However, a stool test may not always pick up a parasite, so there are more specific tests that can be ordered if needed.

Since testing can be expensive, I have created a protocol that can help remove parasites, bacteria and yeast overgrowth from the gut. My Ultimate Gut Support kit contains many of the ingredients from this section. This kit includes digestive enzymes and leaky gut support as well, and is found on my website shop (DrBeckyCampbell.com).

GETTING WELL

One way to get rid of parasites is to create an inhospitable environment for them. To do this, you will need to eliminate sugar and artificial sweeteners from your diet along with dairy and grains.

Instead, consume plant-based foods, increase your fiber intake to help flush out parasites and add the following to your diet, which both fight off parasites and are okay for a low-histamine plan:

- Raw garlic
- Beets
- Pomegranates
- Carrots
- Coconut oil (coconut may not be okay for those with histamine intolerance; as you will see, this food can be found on the Maybe List on page 57)
- Apple cider vinegar (apple cider vinegar may not be okay for those with histamine intolerance, which is why it is also on the Maybe List on page 57)

SUPPLEMENTATION

If you have parasites, you might consider the following supplements:

- Oregano oil
- Clove oil
- Mimosa pudica
- L-glutamine

- Zinc
- Goldenseal
- Black walnut
- Grapefruit seed extract
- Wormwood

CAUSE 5

INFLAMMATORY DIGESTIVE DISEASES

Inflammatory bowel disease (IBD) and other inflammatory digestive diseases are closely linked with issues relating to low DAO, due to the inflammatory effects they have on the body. Histamine levels can also be higher in the gut in those who suffer from inflammatory bowel diseases. The amount of histamine often mirrors the amount of inflammation present.

I want to address a couple of different inflammatory digestive diseases for you.

IBD is a term used to describe chronic inflammatory conditions of the digestive tract. Both Crohn's disease and ulcerative colitis are classified under the term IBD. When you have IBD, you may go through periods when symptoms are severe and experience periods of remission.

While the exact cause of IBD is not known, there are some things that can put you at an increased risk, including poor dietary and lifestyle habits and chronic stress. Having any type of immune system malfunction can also be a risk factor, as an improper immune response can cause the immune system to attack healthy digestive tissue. Having a family history of IBD can also put you at an increased risk of developing it. However, keep in mind that anyone can have IBD, whether it is present in their family or not.

Let's now look at two specific conditions classified under the term IBD.

CROHN'S DISEASE

Crohn's disease is a type of IBD that commonly affects the end of the small bowel and the beginning of the colon. However, it can affect any part of the GI tract anywhere from the mouth to the anus. It's important to know that symptoms of Crohn's disease can vary from person to person, but some of the most common symptoms include the following:

- Urgent need to move the bowels
- Rectal bleeding
- Constipation
- Abdominal pain
- Abdominal cramping
- Diarrhea
- Weight loss
- Loss of appetite
- Fatigue
- Fever

GETTING WELL

When dealing with Crohn's disease, it is important to avoid any foods you are sensitive to. Because no two people will have the exact same food sensitivities, proper testing is key to determine which foods work for you and which foods don't—common culprits include carbonated drinks, alcohol, caffeine, gluten, dairy and grains. By eliminating the foods that are causing inflammation, you can better support your gut.

Eating a nourishing diet is a great way to support your body if you're dealing with this inflammatory condition, and a low-histamine diet can be very beneficial if you are suffering from Crohn's in conjunction with histamine intolerance.

SUPPLEMENTATION

There are some supplements that have been known to help support an inflammatory bowel disease like Crohn's.

Slippery Elm

Slippery elm is great for those with Crohn's disease because it is considered a demulcent, which means it can help protect tissue in the gut and promote tissue healing. It can also help coat the stomach as well as the intestines, so supplementing with slippery elm is a great way to help support overall gut health and to help with any flare-ups.

Probiotics

Probiotics can be helpful for those with Crohn's, but I will talk more about probiotics on page 175, as they can be problematic for some people with histamine intolerance.

Curcumin

One of the strongest anti-inflammatory supplements, curcumin is excellent for reducing overall inflammation and may even be able to reduce certain symptoms associated with Crohn's disease.

L-Glutamine

Along with helping leaky gut, L-glutamine can also be beneficial for those with Crohn's disease because it helps support the intestines.

Omega-3 Fatty Acids

Omega-3 fatty acids contain potent anti-inflammatory properties, which are helpful for those suffering from Crohn's disease.

ULCERATIVE COLITIS

Another type of IBD is ulcerative colitis. This condition is different from Crohn's disease in that it affects the colon or large intestine. Ulcerative colitis is categorized based on the location it affects and may be classified as ulcerative proctitis, proctosig-moiditis, left-sided colitis, pancolitis or acute severe ulcerative colitis.

Symptoms of this inflammatory condition tend to develop more slowly, and they are less likely to come on suddenly. If left untreated, ulcerative colitis can become very serious. Some of the most common symptoms associated with ulcerative colitis include these:

* Weight loss
* Fatigue
* Diarrhea
* Abdominal pain
* Abdominal cramping
* Inability to have a bowel movement despite feeling the sudden urge
* Rectal bleeding and pain

As with Crohn's disease, symptoms will vary from person to person, and some may suffer more than others. Remission is also possible, and you may go into a period of remission for quite a long time before symptoms return.

Diet and lifestyle factors like stress are known to worsen ulcerative colitis, and having an immune system condition can also put you at an increased risk. When your immune system isn't working properly, it may attack healthy digestive tissue as it tries to fight off pathogens. Family history may play a role, but many people who have ulcerative colitis don't have a family history of it.

GETTING WELL

If you suspect you have ulcerative colitis, or you have already been diagnosed, there are some steps you can take to help support your body. A healing diet is the best place to start and if histamine intolerance is something that you deal with on top of ulcerative colitis, then you will want to focus on a low-histamine diet, like the one I will be discussing throughout the rest of this book.

Removing inflammatory and trigger foods is essential, as ulcerative colitis is an inflammatory condition. Some of the most common trigger foods for those with ulcerative colitis include alcohol, caffeine, dairy products, high-fiber foods, nuts, spicy foods, refined sugar, sugar alcohols, artificial sweeteners, beans and raw vegetables. Some people with ulcerative colitis also have a hard time with meat, which is why a low-histamine diet that is high in cooked vegetables may be very beneficial. Also remove gluten, grains and packaged foods from your diet. Enjoy more anti-inflammatory plant-based foods such as low-histamine fruits and vegetables. The supplements discussed for Crohn's disease (page 42) are also beneficial.

Reducing stress is something else that plays a very important role in controlling ulcerative colitis symptoms. Stress and digestive conditions go hand in hand no matter what type of digestive disease you are dealing with. The more able you are to manage and deal with your stress, the better you will feel. Exercise can also be helpful because it helps decrease stress and is excellent for overall health.

CAUSE 6
NUTRIENT DEFICIENCIES

Having a deficiency in certain vitamins or minerals can lead to problems with low DAO, so it is an important potential cause of histamine intolerance. Copper and vitamin C are necessary components of DAO production. Copper and vitamin C help increase DAO function, so having a deficiency can lead to a decrease in DAO or poor DAO function. They can also be helpful for reducing histamine levels, so it is important to rule out a potential deficiency and monitor levels closely. Most people think we need to detox our bodies from copper when what we really need is properly balanced levels.

Vitamin B_6 is important because it helps DAO break down histamine. But while B_6 is vital for supporting DAO, high doses of it can actually destroy bioavailable copper, leaving you with a copper deficiency.

It is important to also test levels of zinc (which has an inverse relationship to copper in the body) and ceruloplasmin (which stores and carries copper in the body) to find out whether a copper deficiency could be a possible underlying cause of your histamine intolerance.

GETTING WELL

If blood tests show that you have a copper deficiency, try including kale, liver, soaked almonds and sesame seeds (if tolerated) in your diet to help support copper levels. These foods are high in copper while also being the lowest histamine of the high copper foods. However, if you notice you are not tolerating these high-copper foods well, find a practitioner who will test you for the other deficiencies discussed earlier.

CAUSE 7
GENETIC MUTATIONS

More and more people are becoming interested in finding out whether they have any type of gene mutation. New DNA and single nucleotide polymorphisms (SNPs) testing have made this much easier.

A little disclaimer here: Genetic testing could open up a can of worms you may not want to know about. Many companies will give you a laundry list of supplements they think you should take based on the SNPs you have, which may not be necessary. However, some mutations potentially lead to an increased risk of histamine intolerance, which is what makes these tests so beneficial.

GENES AND ENZYMES INVOLVED IN HISTAMINE REGULATION

Before I jump into talking about the genetic mutations that are often linked to histamine intolerance, I want to briefly talk about the different genes and enzymes and what they do.

MTHFR

The MTHFR gene is needed to make the enzyme methylenetetrahydrofolate reductase. This enzyme is essential for processing amino acids and converting homocysteine into methionine. It also plays a very important role when it comes to methylation and removing toxins from the body. Histamine needs methylation in order to be processed and eliminated from the body.

HNMT

HNMT is a gene that is needed for processing histamine. It also plays a role in regulating histamine and breaking it down.

SAMe

S-Adenosyl-L-methionine (SAMe) is a cofactor of HNMT and is naturally made in the body. It is important for the formation, activation and breakdown of various hormones, proteins and drugs. Many people take a SAMe supplement to help with anxiety, depression, PMS, premenstrual dysphoric disorder and fibromyalgia when they may not make enough SAMe on their own.

MAO

MAO is an enzyme responsible for breaking down histamine.

DAO

DAO, the enzyme we have been talking a lot about so far, is essential for breaking down built-up histamine in the body.

N-acetyltransferase 2N-acetyltransferase 2 (NAT2) works to deactivate carcinogens and hydrazine drugs, which may be used as a treatment for certain cancers.

GENETIC LINKS TO HISTAMINE INTOLERANCE

HNMT, a gene that is critical for processing histamine, requires SAMe as a cofactor, and SAMe requires a functioning MTHFR enzyme in order to be produced. It's a domino effect: When the MTHFR gene is mutated, SAMe production may not work as it should, which can then disrupt the HNMT gene. This can slow the removal of histamine from the body, causing the symptoms linked to histamine intolerance. Having an MTHFR gene mutation can also decrease the body's ability to methylate properly. Methylation is important for removing toxins and built-up histamine from the body.

DAO, MAO, HNMT and NAT2 are essential for processing histamine. If any of these is mutated in any way, it can interfere with removing histamine from the body. This interference can lead to histamine intolerance and the symptoms associated with it.

TESTING FOR GENETIC MUTATIONS

To test for genetic mutations using SNP testing, the 23andMe test is the standard test as of this writing. While they do not give you a list of all the genetic SNPs listed earlier, you can put your raw data given to you by 23andMe into a third-party company and they can give you a genetic report to determine which gene mutations could be relevant to your health issues. Be wary of companies that prescribe you a bunch of supplements based on these findings. We only know the tip of the iceberg when it comes to genetic testing and what it all means. Having a genetic SNP does not mean you have an actual health condition. I prefer companies like StrateGene (http://go.strategene.org/genetic-analysis) from Dr. Ben Lynch for accurate results you can trust.

Knowing whether you have one of these gene mutations is the first step in uncovering a potential genetic susceptibility to histamine intolerance. If you do have a genetic mutation, all is not lost. There are many things you can do to start feeling better.

GETTING WELL

If you have an MTHFR gene mutation, you can:

- Consume natural folate and stay away from folic acid (a great source of folate is dark leafy vegetables, which are also low in histamine);
- Support digestive health issues, such as leaky gut and irritable bowel syndrome;
- Try to manage stress and anxiety with mindfulness training, prayer or qigong;
- Boost your body's natural ability to detoxify itself by exercising, staying hydrated, dry-brushing your skin and consuming lots of low-histamine vegetables.

CAUSE 8
CERTAIN MEDICATIONS

Certain medications, such as NSAIDs, antidepressants, immune modulators, anti-arrhythmics, antihistamines and histamine blockers can all lead to low DAO. Many people are confused to see histamine blockers such as Pepcid, Zantac and Tagamet on the list of medications that can lead to low DAO. However, antihistamines can indeed lead to a depletion of DAO in the body, making histamine intolerance worse.

NEXT STEPS

Having histamine intolerance can be overwhelming and confusing. However, there are a number of things you can do to feel better and get your histamine levels under control. Before I dive into the things you can do, I want to stress that the whole body must be supported when treating histamine intolerance. If just one body system is left unsupported and out of balance, your attempts to get the histamine under control may not work.

While you may work very hard on correcting your diet, making healthier lifestyle choices and supporting other areas of the body are just as important. For example, while you may be eating better, avoiding high-histamine foods and reducing stress, you may not be correcting an undiagnosed gut infection. Without doing so, you won't feel as good as you could. This is why I stress the importance of working with a functional-medicine practitioner or taking part in my Histamine Intolerance Online Course at DrBeckyCampbell.com to uncover all of your triggers and support your whole body, so that you can enjoy the absolute best outcome.

GETTING WELL

Review your medication history with a skilled and open-minded practitioner to see whether a certain medication is triggering histamine intolerance and what can be done about it. Do not stop or start any medication without the help of a practitioner.

Three
THE 4-PHASE
HISTAMINE RESET PLAN

PHASE 1
ELIMINATE

FIND YOUR ROOT CAUSE

A big part of treating histamine intolerance is finding the root cause. Some individuals may have one, while others may have a couple. Did you identify your root causes as you read through Chapter 2? That chapter will help you determine what may be causing your symptoms and how to better get your histamine intolerance under control.

REMOVE HIGH-HISTAMINE AND INFLAMMATORY FOODS FOR 1 TO 3 MONTHS

If you have histamine intolerance or suspect that you do, the first step is to remove high-histamine and inflammatory foods from your diet for 1 to 3 months. Don't worry, I have detailed exactly how to do this in the next section. You will be removing these foods in one or two phases, depending on how you respond. By breaking it down into two separate phases, you will find the diet to be less intimidating. It also makes it easier to pinpoint exactly what may be causing your symptoms.

During this phase, it is very important to keep a food diary (download link on page 61) as a way to help determine which foods are triggering immediate symptoms. It is also essential to keep an eye on your general level of inflammation and stress.

Let me explain the concept of bucket theory. The idea is that once your body's "bucket" is filled with histamine, you will see a reaction. Until that tipping point, you could be symptom-free. More importantly, when you concentrate on low-inflammatory foods, it can allow you to take in more histamine without a reaction. In addition to high-histamine and high-inflammatory foods, things like stress, environmental toxins, hormone levels, drugs and nutrient deficiencies can fill our histamine bucket.

This is why an anti-inflammatory diet, stress-relieving activities and getting to the root cause of the histamine intolerance are key. The guidelines you will follow in this plan are mostly a Paleo-type diet (i.e., one that relies on low-inflammatory foods) with the removal of high-histamine foods. Occasionally, you will see I call for a low-histamine cheese like raw mozzarella, which is not technically Paleo. But it's something you can try—see how you react to it.

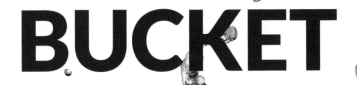

OUR HISTAMINE BUCKET

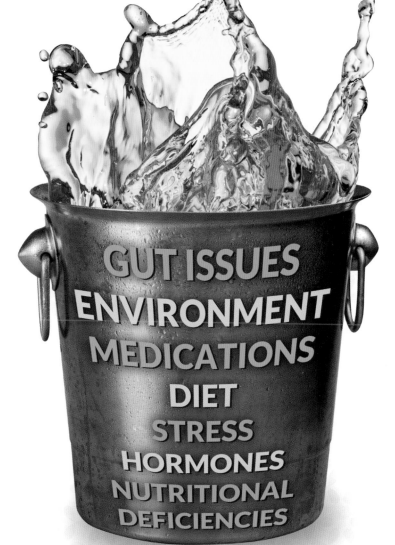

GUT ISSUES
ENVIRONMENT
MEDICATIONS
DIET
STRESS
HORMONES
NUTRITIONAL
DEFICIENCIES

NO ALLERGY REQUIRED

The reason I only recommend having raw mozzarella is because raw dairy is known to have less of an inflammatory effect on the body than conventional dairy. Follow a low-inflammatory and low-histamine plan and use the tools we talked about to keep stress at bay, and you will keep your baseline of inflammation low. You will also keep your ability to eat some foods that contain histamine much higher!

During these two phases, you will be eliminating high-histamine foods as well as some histamine liberators and DAO-blocking foods. High-histamine foods are foods that contain a lot of histamine, so they are most often very problematic for those with histamine intolerance. Histamine liberators are foods that are not high in histamine, but they cause histamine release in the body. DAO-blocking foods are, as the name implies, foods that block DAO, the enzyme needed to break down histamine.

Keep in mind that if you are suffering from histamine intolerance, it doesn't mean you will have to keep these foods out of your diet forever. The low-histamine diet may be a temporary measure until your histamine and DAO levels stabilize and you start to feel better. Plus I am going to give you other methods to help your body tolerate these foods as well. However, you may find that you have to keep some foods out of your diet forever.

I always stress to my patients how important it is to stay positive during this elimination period! Your histamine and DAO levels could normalize faster than you think. Just keep moving through the low-histamine diet and keep a detailed food journal. The more you track, the better your results.

CONSIDER A LOWER-PROTEIN, HIGHER-VEGGIE DIET

After you follow the low-histamine diet, you may be wondering what you should be doing long term. I recommend a lower-protein (notice I did not say low), higher-vegetable diet. Why? Because histamine is made from amino acids, which are derived from proteins. When you consume a diet high in protein, you will naturally be consuming more foods high in histamine. During the diet and after, I recommend 3 to 4 ounces (84 to 112 g) of clean protein and two or three servings of vegetables per meal.

REMOVE COFFEE AND CAFFEINE FROM YOUR DIET

Okay, don't hate me for saying this, but removing coffee and caffeine from your diet is important when you are dealing with histamine intolerance. While caffeine doesn't directly trigger the release of histamine, it can block DAO, making it difficult to break down built-up histamine. This includes coffee, tea, chocolate, coffee- or chocolate-flavored ice cream, hot chocolate, sodas and decaf coffee (which still contains a small amount of caffeine).

REPLACE TOXIC HOME AND PERSONAL CARE PRODUCTS

Although we have already talked about removing certain toxins from your home, including foods and certain medications, there are some other toxins we need to talk about. These toxins are found in your home, and you may not even be aware that they pose health risks. I'm talking about cleaning sprays, soaps and laundry detergent.

HIGH-HISTAMINE, HISTAMINE-LIBERATING & DAO-ENZYME-BLOCKING FOODS

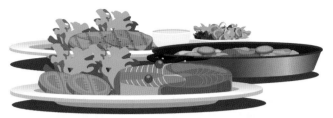

In addition to high-histamine foods, there are also histamine-liberating foods and DAO-blocking foods that should be avoided. You will see some of these foods in the No List and some of them in the Maybe List (page 57).

High-Histamine Foods

Aged Cheese: including goat cheese
Citrus Fruits: (see exceptions on page 57 in the Maybe List)
Canned & Cured Meats: bacon, pepperoni, salami, lunch meat, canned meats & hot dogs
Dried Fruits: apricots, dates, figs, prunes & raisins
Fermented Foods: kefir, Kombucha, sauerkraut, soy sauce, vinegar (see pages 57 & 170 about vinegars)
Fermented Alcohol: beer, champagne, wine especially
Legumes: beans, lentils, peanuts & soy
Nuts: cashews & walnuts
Processed Foods: all types, preservatives are high in histamine
Soured Foods: buttermilk, sour cream, sour milk, etc.
Smoked Fish & these Species of Fish: anchovies, mackerel, mahi-mahi, sardines, tuna, fish sauce
Veggies: avocados, eggplant, spinach & tomatoes
Vinegar-Containing Foods: olives, pickles (see pages 57 & 170 about vinegars)

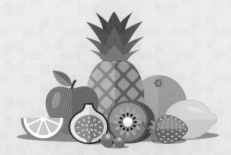

Histamine-Liberating Foods
These foods can be low in histamine themselves, but can help release histamine in the body.

Alcohol	Nuts	Strawberries
Bananas	Papaya	Tomatoes
Chocolate	Pineapple	Wheat germ
Cow's milk	Shellfish	Many artificial preservatives and dyes

DAO-Enzyme-Blocking Foods
These foods can block the enzyme responsible for breaking down histamine in the body.

Alcohol
Black tea
Energy drinks
Green tea
Mate tea

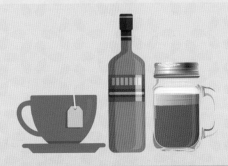

All of these can cause issues for a handful of reasons. For one, they often contain fragrance, which can cause endocrine disruption in the body. Some products also release volatile organic compounds (VOCs). VOCs are commonly found in aerosol sprays, air fresheners, detergents, oven cleaners and rug cleaners. These VOCs have been shown to lead to respiratory issues, headaches and allergic reactions, which is the last thing we want when trying to get histamine under control.

To help avoid the toxic products in your home, I recommend making your own cleaning products as much as possible. You can make your own all-purpose cleaner using castile soap and a few drops of pure essential oils.

As for dish detergent and laundry detergent, I recommend choosing natural options that are free from fragrance and toxic chemicals. You can find clean and toxin-free products on the Environmental Working Group website (www.ewg.org). The more you can reduce your toxin exposure, the better you will feel. Remember, getting histamine intolerance under control means supporting the entire body.

PHASE 2
SUPPORT THE LIVER

THE IMPORTANCE OF YOUR LIVER

Liver support is critical when you are dealing with histamine intolerance, and the relationship can play out in a few different ways. For example, having too much histamine can lead to liver-enzyme changes, harming the organ. And having liver dysfunction can lead to histamine intolerance.

The liver also plays a major role in removing toxins from the body, so great liver health supports great overall health. For this reason, it is important to support your liver. Here are some ways you can do that.

EPSOM SALT BATHS

I love recommending Epsom salt baths. They are a natural way to support the liver through detoxification, and they can also be very relaxing (remember, reducing stress is a big part of controlling histamine intolerance). The magnesium sulfate in Epsom salt is what helps remove built-up toxins from the body. You can add a couple of drops of pure lavender essential oil to your bath to make it even more relaxing.

CASTOR OIL PACKS

Castor oil has long been used to help detoxify the body, but drinking the oil can lead to some dangerous side effects. For this reason, I recommend castor oil packs, which you can place over your liver to help support liver function. I love the starter kit from Heritage Store (heritagestore.com), as it includes everything you need.

INFRARED SAUNAS

Infrared saunas are a fabulous tool for anyone with symptoms of histamine intolerance. They can help with stress management and provide the detoxification benefits just like moderate exercise. This is because sweating helps us release stored toxins. The skin is a major organ of elimination, and infrared saunas are particularly helpful in releasing toxic contaminants like mercury and lead. They heat your tissues several inches deep, enhancing your natural metabolic processes, improving your circulation and oxygenating your tissues. Infrared saunas also improve heart function, boost well-being and reduce depression and feelings of anger. I recommend enjoying an infrared sauna two or three times per week.

LIVER FUNCTIONS

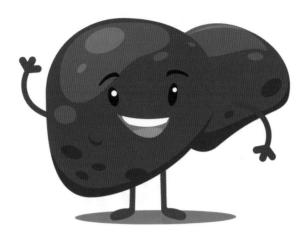

Helps convert T4 (inactive form of thyroid hormone) to T3 (active, usable form of thyroid hormone) to be used in the body

Breaks down nutrients from food to produce energy in the body

Removes bacteria from the blood to help your body fight infection

Removes toxins from the body

Stores mineral, vitamins and sugar for your body to use

Helps balance hormone levels

Creates cholesterol for hormone production and tissue healing

SUPPLEMENTS

Supplements to support the liver include milk thistle; N-Acetyl-L-Cysteine (NAC), and others listed in my Optimal Reset Liver Love supplement list on page 176.

PHASE 3
GO DEEPER

HEAL THE GUT

As a functional-medicine doctor who works with patients with histamine intolerance and thyroid disease, I know how important healing the gut is. In fact, it may just be the most important step you take, as having an imbalance in the gut can lead to an imbalance somewhere else. This is even more important for those who have any type of immune system imbalance, as roughly 70 percent of the immune system resides in the gut.

Gut imbalances have been linked to autoimmune disease, anxiety, depression, skin issues and hormonal imbalances. Having an imbalance in the bacteria in the gut can also lead to things like SIBO and candida, which are underlying causes of histamine intolerance. As we have previously discussed, certain bacteria in the gut can produce histamine, leading to a buildup of histamine in the body while also impairing DAO function, the enzyme needed to break down histamine.

There are countless reasons why we need to support the gut, and many of these reasons directly affect histamine intolerance. Let's take a look at some of the ways you can support gut health.

TEST FOR GUT INFECTIONS

Testing for gut infections is relatively simple. Work with a functional-medicine practitioner to get specific testing and a specific treatment plan for your situation. You can also find out the exact tests you need to uncover your underlying causes, a detailed test interpretation guide and specific protocol based on your test results in my Histamine Intolerance Online Program, found on my website at DrBeckyCampbell.com.

TEST FOR NUTRIENT DEFICIENCIES

As already mentioned, nutrient deficiencies can predispose you to histamine intolerance, so it is important to get tested. If you are deficient in something, try to find high-quality food sources for that nutrient.

WATCH YOUR TOXIC LOAD

Toxins can be found everywhere we turn, but there are many we can avoid. Things like NSAIDs, alcohol and caffeine can all be very hard on the gut. Chronic stress and too much exercise can also pose a problem. Where can you reduce toxins in your life to help support your gut health?

SUPPORT THE HPA AXIS

Because stress is a big histamine trigger, supporting the adrenal glands is essential to combating histamine intolerance symptoms and lowering inflammation. The adrenal glands are responsible for producing key hormones that help the body control blood sugar, blood pressure, electrolyte levels and sex hormones. They also help you cope with physical and emotional stress. Any imbalance can lead to adrenal fatigue and burnout. Adaptogenic herbs like ashwagandha can be helpful, as they help support adrenal health, balance hormone levels and help you feel calmer and more centered.

To support the adrenal glands, I highly recommend meditation and visualization. Meditation switches off the genes related to inflammation, while visualization can quickly change your mind-set, lower stress when you are experiencing histamine-related symptoms, and aid the healing process (though be sure to always seek out the appropriate medical care in an emergency and when needed).

I also recommend the dried urine test for comprehensive hormones to my patients, so we can measure their stress hormones and sex hormone levels. This is one of the many helpful tools we use in my Histamine Intolerance Online Course, found on my website.

IMPROVE YOUR SLEEP HABITS

I recommend improving your sleep habits as much as possible. I understand that this can be challenging. Sleep is essential for stress management and supporting the adrenal glands, so try to get at least eight hours of uninterrupted sleep per night and rest when you feel like your body is craving it.

If you already suffer from adrenal dysfunction, you may need more than eight hours of sleep each night, so take this into account when deciding what time your healthiest bedtime might be. Here are some easy methods to optimize your sleep cycle:

- Keep all screens out of the bedroom
- Make sure your bedroom is as dark, cool and quiet as possible
- Aim to wind down during the evening, two hours before your actual bedtime by doing some light chores
- Read poetry, a novel or other nonstimulating literature before you fall asleep and stay away from news, studying and business-related reading material at this time

SUPPLEMENTS FOR HISTAMINE INTOLERANCE

While some supplements combat deficiencies, others can specifically help with histamine intolerance. For a list of the supplements I recommend, check out the supplement guide (page 175), where you'll find some of my favorite options and links to the actual products.

PHASE 4
REINTRODUCE

During phase 4 of this plan, you can reintroduce certain high-histamine foods. With any food you reintroduce, try it for three days straight and track any symptoms that you experience in a symptom tracker.

DOWNLOAD SYMPTOM TRACKER

http://bit.ly/HITtracker

Try to add as much detail as possible, and use a grading system (1 to 10) to record their severity.

If you do experience any symptoms, eliminate the food right away. If you have gone through phase 3, start by adding foods from phase 3 back into your diet one at a time. Then move on to foods from phase 1. We'll be covering these foods in the next chapter.

It is important to know that you may never be able to eat certain high-histamine foods, even if your body is able to tolerate histamine better. I can eat a lot of these foods now, but I can't eat them all, and I notice the same with my patients. However, everyone is different, so test each of the foods one by one and keep a very detailed food journal to identify what will and won't work for your body.

Four

DR. BECKY'S **4-PHASE LOW-HISTAMINE DIET**

Now that you are ready to begin a low-histamine diet, I want to explain how it works.

The diet focuses on eliminating foods that people most often respond to the worst, rather than eliminating all high-histamine foods at once. This makes the diet a little less intimidating and easier to jump into.

You will find a list of foods you can eat freely (the Yes List), foods to try (the Maybe List) and foods that you should avoid (the No List). See how you do as you go through the phases. You can eliminate these foods if you react poorly at any time. As I've mentioned, you will want to keep a food diary to be able to pinpoint any foods you may be reacting to.

THE YES/NO/MAYBE LIST

Here is how this list is broken down.

THE YES LIST: YOUR BEST FRIENDS

As the name implies, the foods on the Yes List are going to be your "best friends" during this phase. They should be safe for everyone with histamine intolerance. So if you do have a reaction to these foods, it is most likely because of an issue that is not related to histamine intolerance.

THE NO LIST: THE USUAL SUSPECTS

The items on the No List are foods that most people with histamine intolerance react to. These are foods you may never be able to eat without feeling unwell, or you may be able to add them to your diet after healing your gut. However, in the beginning, it's best to completely eliminate these foods.

THE MAYBE LIST: SNEAKY SIDEKICKS

The Maybe List contains foods that may or may not cause an immediate problem for those with histamine intolerance. In fact, they may not bother you at all, but they may bother some, producing subtler symptoms.

You can either choose to stay away from these foods, or try them one at a time and keep a detailed food journal to log the effects. Keep in mind that if you react to a food, you may experience symptoms for up to a few days afterward, so a food journal is essential if you want to identify which foods you can tolerate and which foods you cannot.

DR. BECKY'S LOW HISTAMINE PLAN
PHASE 1

YES FOODS
(EAT FREELY)

PROTEIN
(must be fresh or frozen)

Beef
Bison
Chicken
Duck
Elk
Lamb
Pasture-Raised Eggs (whites must be cooked)
Pheasant
Pork
Rabbit
Seafood (must be very fresh)
Turkey
Venison
Wild Boar

FRUITS
(must be fresh or frozen)

Apples
Apricots
Blackberries
Blueberries
Cherries
Exotic Fruit (star fruit, quince)
Grapes
Melon
Pears

FATS
Extra-Virgin Olive Oil
Ghee
Grass-Fed Butter
Coconut Oil

SWEETENER
Blackstrap Molasses
Honey (local is best)
Maple Syrup/Maple Sugar
Coconut Sugar

FLOURS
Arrowroot
Cassava
Coconut flour
Tapioca

VEGETABLES
Anise/Fennel Root
Artichoke
Arugula
Asparagus
Beets
Bell Peppers
Bok Choy
Broccoli
Brussels Sprouts
Cabbage
Carrots
Cauliflower
Celery
Collard Greens
Cucumber
Garlic
Green Beans
Greens (beet, mustard, turnip)
Jicama
Kale
Leeks
Lettuce (bibb, butter, red)
Onions/Shallots
Parsnips
Rutabaga
Sweet Potatoes/Yams
Swiss Chard
Turnip
Watercress
Zucchini

OTHERS
Celtic or Himalayan Sea Salt
Leafy Herbs
Pepper
White Tea and Herbal Teas

NO FOODS
(DO NOT EAT)

PROTEIN
Anything that is in the Yes Protein List that is not fresh and/or leftovers

FRUITS
Avocado
Citrus
Dried Fruit (Apricots, Prunes, Dates, Figs, Raisins)
Strawberries
Tomato
Banana

VEGETABLES
Eggplant
Spinach

NUTS
(highest in histamine)

Cashews
Walnuts

ADDITIONAL FOODS
(not all high in histamine but may cause inflammation)

Alcohol (especially red wine)
Beans
Chocolate
Cinnamon
Dairy
Fermented Foods
Gluten
Grains
Peanuts
Soy

VINEGARS
All Vinegars (except gluten-free distilled white vinegar and apple cider vinegar, which are the lowest in histamine)

Vinegar-Containing Products (e.g., olives, mustard, ketchup, mayo)

SPICES
Anise
Cinnamon
Cloves
Curry Powder
Paprika/Cayenne
Nutmeg
Seasoning packets with restrictive ingredients
Foods labeled "with spices"

MAYBE FOODS
(EAT MODERATELY)

FRUITS
Raspberries
Kiwi
Lemon
Lime
Mango
Nectarine
Papaya
Peach
Plum

VEGETABLES
Mushrooms
Peas
Pumpkin
Squash

NUTS
Soaked Almonds, Pecans, Pistachio
Soaked Brazil and Pine Nuts

OTHER
Apple Cider Vinegar
Coconut Products (coconut milk, coconut butter, shredded coconut)
Dried Herbs/Spices
Gelatin/Collagen
Gluten-Free Distilled White Vinegar
Yeast

SEED AND SEED BUTTERS
Flax, Sesame, Sunflower
Pumpkin

FLOURS
(most people do ok with these but check your tolerance)

Almond Flour

OTHER FOODS TO AVOID

Although not all of these foods are high in histamine, they are inflammatory and are best avoided for optimum health. They include gluten, grains, dairy, refined sugar and soy.

I follow a mostly Paleo-style diet, and I recommend that my patients do as well, because the diet removes these inflammatory foods and focuses on replacing them with low-inflammatory options.

HISTAMINE HEALING FOODS

Many foods are great for supporting histamine intolerance and helping reduce inflammation, which is a big part of getting this condition under control. Other foods specifically work to help control the amount of histamine in the body. Let's take a look at some of the top foods for histamine intolerance.

GINGER

Ginger helps reduce inflammation in the body and is great for digestive health. It acts as an all-natural antihistamine and tastes delicious in stir-fries and smoothies.

PEPPERMINT

Peppermint contains flavonoids that may be able to inhibit histamine from mast cells. Some people even enjoy peppermint during allergy season to help better control their symptoms. You can try making a homemade peppermint tea or add fresh mint to recipes like tabbouleh.

THYME

Thyme is another herb that is beneficial for people with histamine intolerance. It is rich in vitamin C and even contains some antimicrobial health benefits, making it great for immune health.

POMEGRANATES

Pomegranates are excellent for fighting inflammation and are very high in antioxidants. Pomegranate juice is really delicious. The fruit can also be added to a smoothie to help combat inflammation.

ARUGULA

Arugula is an impressive anti-inflammatory food and is even thought to have some anticancer benefits. Arugula makes a great addition to any salad. You can mix arugula with any other dark leafy vegetable for added health benefits and extra flavor.

ARTICHOKES

Artichokes are rich in luteolin, a flavonoid that helps stabilize mast cells. Remember, we want to stabilize mast cells so they don't release excess amounts of histamine and cause histamine buildup in the body.

WATERCRESS

Watercress is another anti-inflammatory veggie that works well to help prevent too much histamine from being released in the body when we are exposed to allergens. Watercress also tastes great when added to salads if you like a spicier flavor.

ONIONS

Onions are a staple in so many recipes due to their unique flavor. They have a way of dressing up just about any savory dish and they hold some impressive health benefits. Onions may be able to inhibit histamine release and help lower histamine levels as well. Try adding chopped onions to meat-based dishes or even to scrambled eggs or omelets. You can also add onions to salads for an extra kick.

GARLIC

Garlic, another favorite addition to savory dishes and an antioxidant powerhouse, may be able to prevent histamine release from mast cells. Garlic tastes great in meat-based dishes or with steamed, baked or sautéed vegetables.

DAO ENZYME-BOOSTING FOODS, PALEO STYLE

Because one of the most important jobs of the DAO enzyme is to break down histamine, it is important to eat foods that are proven to give it a boost. Some of these foods are on the Maybe List, so keep an eye out for how they may affect you.

Protein:

- Grass-fed liver (if you can tolerate it)
- Pasture-raised chicken
- Pasture-raised eggs
- Salmon (wild-caught and fresh or frozen only)
- Sardines (fresh only)

Fruits and Veggies:

- Beet greens
- Broccoli
- Chard
- Collard greens

Nuts and Seeds:

- Almonds
- Pistachios
- Pumpkin seeds

QUERCETIN-RICH FOODS

One of the reasons why onions can be so helpful for people with histamine intolerance is that they are high in quercetin, which helps lower histamine. Quercetin is a plant flavanol that works to reduce allergic responses in the body while also supporting the immune system.

A chart showing quercetin-rich foods appears on page 60.

HIGH-QUERCETIN/ LOW-HISTAMINE FOODS

FRUITS

Grapes

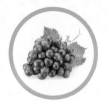
Apples

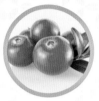
Cranberries

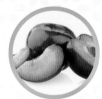
Black Plums

Blueberries

Chokeberries

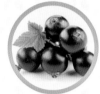
Black Currants

Cherries

VEGGIES

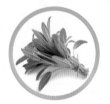
Sage

Herbs

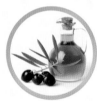
Olive Oil

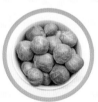
Cruciferous Veggies

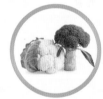
Broccoli

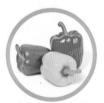
Peppers

Red Leaf Lettuce

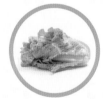
Romaine Lettuce

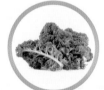
Raw Kale

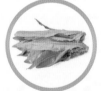
Chicory Greens

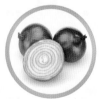
Raw Red Onion

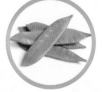
Snap Peas

Raw Asparagus

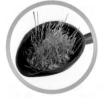
Sprouts

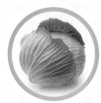
Cabbage

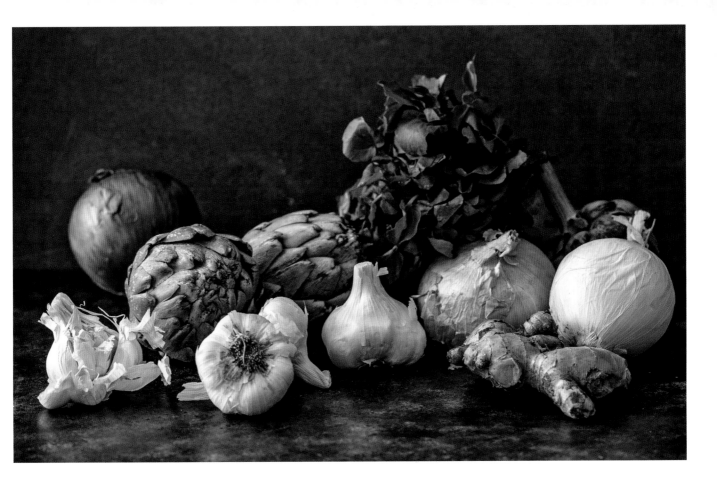

LOW-HISTAMINE DIET TIPS

- Cook your own meals as much as possible.
- Eat the freshest food possible (caught or picked fresh or frozen).
- Record everything you eat in a detailed daily food diary (download a food diary at http://bit.ly/HITjournal).
- Record the times and dates of any uncomfortable symptoms for comparison (download a symptom tracker log at http://bit.ly/HITtracker).
- Avoid junk food and anything processed (especially canned foods).
- Freeze leftovers immediately if possible instead of storing in the refrigerator.
- Use fresh herbs instead of dried herbs when possible.

Use your Instant Pot® when possible to avoid longer cook times. The longer foods take to cook, the more histamine they release.

WHAT TO EAT IN EACH PHASE

Here is how you will eat during the 4-Phase Low-Histamine Diet.

WHAT TO EAT IN PHASE 1

During phase 1, feel free to eat any or all of the foods on the Yes List and the foods on the Maybe List in moderation. Foods on the No List should be completely avoided. You will also notice additional foods to eliminate that are not high in histamine but are inflammatory. See page 48 for more information.

WHAT TO EAT IN PHASE 2

While you're in phase 2, maintain the diet you've developed during phase 1 while adding the activities that cleanse and support your liver. As you'll remember, these include the following:

- Four weeks of the Optimal Reset Liver Love supplement
- Epsom salt baths
- Castor oil packs
- Infrared saunas

See page 52 for more information.

WHAT TO EAT IN PHASE 3

If you are still having symptoms once you've completed phases 1 and 2, you will need to continue to eliminate more foods so you can uncover which foods are triggering your symptoms. Try eliminating the following foods one at a time, while keeping a detailed journal of your symptoms:

- All citrus fruits (including lemon and lime)
- All nuts and seeds (nut milks, nut butters and nut flours; find more information about flours on page 66)
- All vinegars
- Coconut products
- Collagen
- Dried herbs and spices
- Egg whites
- Gelatin
- Kefir
- Kiwis
- Mangoes
- Mushrooms
- Nectarines
- Papayas
- Peaches
- Peas
- Plums
- Pork
- Pumpkins
- Squash
- Yeast

See page 54 for more information.

WHAT TO EAT IN PHASE 4

In phase 4, you will work to reintroduce certain high-histamine foods. Begin by adding one food at a time from phase 3 for three days. Eliminate it if you start to notice any old symptoms returning, and note those symptoms in your journal. Then move on to the foods you eliminated in phase 1 and do the same. Don't forget to make a list of every single food you do and don't react to for later reference. See page 55 for more information.

BUILD YOUR PLATE

FOR BOTH LUNCH AND DINNER, SERVE 3 TO 4 OUNCES
(84 TO 112 G) OF MEAT AND TWO VEGETABLE SIDES.

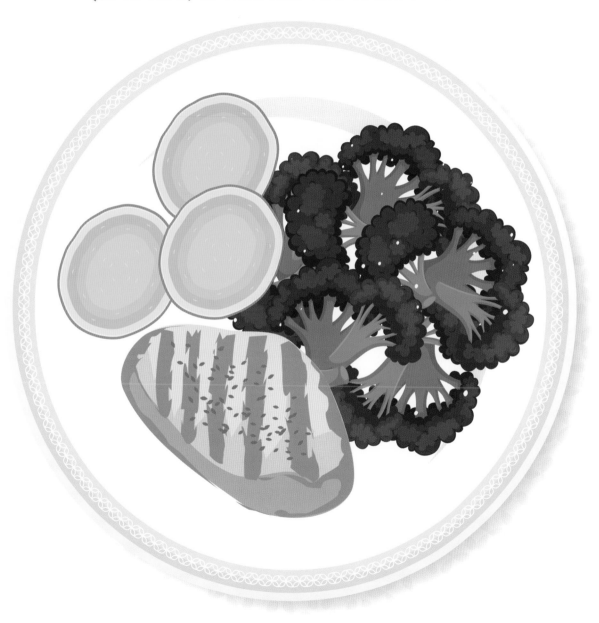

Five

DR. BECKY'S
LOW-HISTAMINE RECIPES

COOKING WITH AN INSTANT POT®

I love cooking with my Instant Pot. Not only does it cut down on cooking and cleanup time, but it is also great for those with histamine intolerance. Because cooking time is usually reduced with the Instant Pot, you decrease the chance of histamine buildup, especially when you are cooking meat. It is also great for making low-histamine bone broth. Instead of making bone broth in 24 hours, you can make it in 2 hours and then freeze it right away, significantly reducing the amount of histamine in the broth.

Although not every recipe in this section uses an Instant Pot, you can use the appliance to cook just about anything, from sautés to broths, soups, stews, vegetables and even hard-boiled eggs. There are different settings you can use to make your dish both perfectly delicious and low in histamine.

FOOD-PREP TIPS

Many individuals with histamine intolerance react poorly to leftover foods. So you will need to get used to preparing food and freezing it immediately when trying to avoid high-histamine foods. However, there are many foods you can prepare ahead of time and store for a few days in the refrigerator. Also, not everyone responds badly to leftovers. This is something to test out to see how you respond—one of the biggest challenges about eating for histamine intolerance is making everything fresh, so it's worth experimenting.

In this section, I explain which foods are best frozen ahead of time and which foods are safe to make and keep in the refrigerator.

FROZEN PATTIES

Once I realized I could take ground chicken, turkey, lamb, bison and grass-fed beef and make it into patties to freeze, dealing with my low-histamine diet got a lot easier. I include recipes for frozen patties later in the book. I recommend making and freezing them weekly so that you can take them out daily to use.

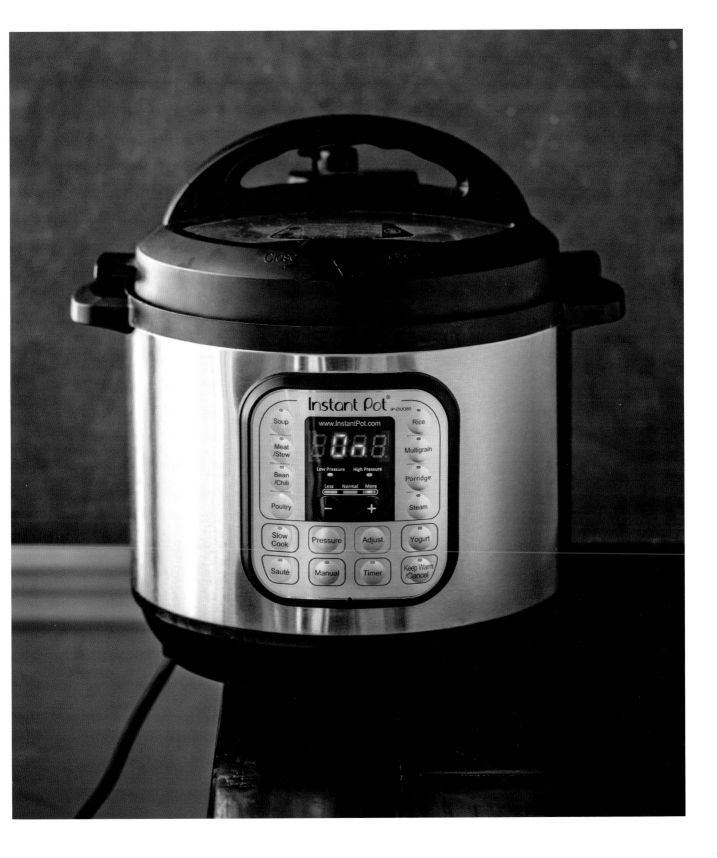

CHICKEN TENDERLOIN

I like to buy a package of chicken tenderloin and divide it between baggies, with two or three tenderloins per bag. These are easy to defrost in the morning and cook for lunch. You can add them to salads or wraps.

COLLARD GREEN WRAPS

Collard green wraps can be made ahead of time and stored in the refrigerator for use during the week.

LOWER-HISTAMINE MAYONNAISE

This should be okay to make ahead of time and use for about three days (see the recipe on page 68). Again, you will need to test this and see how you respond. This is another reason it is so important to keep a food journal.

PORTIONING OUT VEGGIES

This is a great time-saving trick. Simply portion out your pre-cooked veggies and place them in baggies for future use.

LEFTOVER VEGGIES

If you're not sensitive to leftover foods, feel free to warm and serve leftover vegetables from the night before. Not everyone can do this, but it's worth experimenting to find out how you tolerate vegetables that have been stored overnight.

SOURCING AND MAKING YOUR OWN FLOURS

In the recipes, I list a number of different types of flour, including these:

- Cassava or tapioca flour
- Almond flour
- Other types of nut flour
- Tigernut flour
- Coconut flour

Some of these can be made at home in the kitchen, whereas others are easy to pick up online or at a health food store.

Cassava and Tapioca Flours

Cassava flour is gluten-, grain- and nut-free, as well as Paleo. It is very mild and neutral in flavor, as well as soft and powdery. When it comes to gluten-free flour alternatives, it is the most similar to wheat flour, making it extremely useful in baking. It's a good source of vitamin C. You can find it both online and in stores, and as it becomes more popular, it's becoming easier to source. You can also make your own, but you'll need to grate it, dry it in the oven or in a dehydrator, then mill it with a mortar, which can be a little time-consuming.

Tapioca flour is a starch extracted from the cassava root and can be used as a thickener as well as a wheat-flour replacement, but it does have slightly different properties to straight cassava flour.

Almond Flour

Almond flour is the safest of the nut flours for people with histamine intolerance, but you'll want to make sure you can tolerate it before using it more than just occasionally. You can make fresh almond flour using a coffee grinder or high-speed blender, or you can buy it either online or offline. Freshly made is best.

Other Types of Nut Flour

I don't recommend using other types of nut flour available for purchase, as they are generally poorly tolerated and may have been stored for a long time before they reach your kitchen, adding fuel to the fire.

Tigernut Flour

Tigernuts are actually not a nut, as the name may imply. Tigernuts are small root vegetables that can be ground up into another wonderful flour for antihistamine cooking and baking. It is high in fiber, iron, potassium, protein, magnesium, zinc and vitamins E and C. It has been used in Africa for millennia. Its flavor naturally lends itself well to sweet dishes, but it can also be used for flavor balancing in salads and other savory dishes. It can be sourced both online and offline.

Coconut Flour

Coconut flour is a soft flour made from dried coconut meat. It's rich in protein, fiber and fat, making it filling. It can be useful for losing weight and supporting healthy digestion, thanks to its high nutrient density and medium chain fatty acid content, which is stable under high temperatures. It is very absorbent, dense and dry, so it's best to stick with the less-is-more concept when using it. Saying that, it's more economical than almond flour, is low-carb and adds a very nice flavor to sweet dishes. Coconut flour is now readily available both online and in stores, and it keeps well.

LOWER–HISTAMINE MAYONNAISE

Mayonnaise is something I never wanted to give up. I have a few variations of this recipe so that most people will be able to tolerate it with no problem.

MAKES 1 CUP (220 G)

1 large pasture-raised egg

1½ tbsp (20 g) mustard made with distilled white vinegar (such as Annie's brand)

1 cup (240 ml) extra-light tasting olive oil

½ tsp sea salt

Place the egg, mustard, oil and salt in a Mason jar and stick an emulsion blender all the way to the bottom. Once the bottom portion is emulsified, slowly bring the blender up and blend until the next portion is emulsified, going up and down as necessary to create a homogenous mixture. Repeat this process until the mixture is creamy throughout, 1 to 2 minutes.

PHASE 3: If egg whites cause an issue, try using 2 large pasture-raised egg yolks instead of a whole egg. If you still cannot tolerate this, remove this item completely.

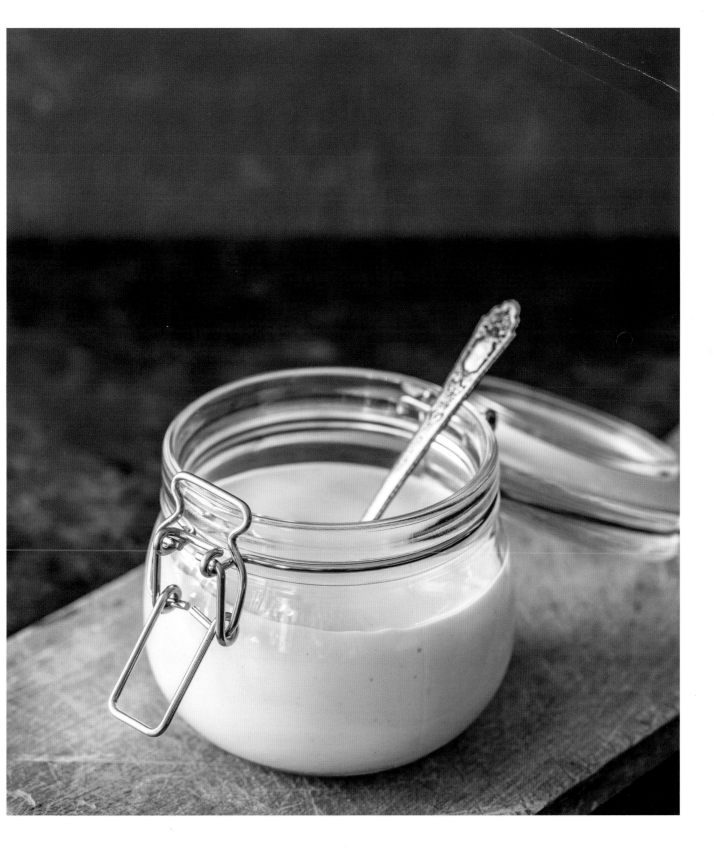

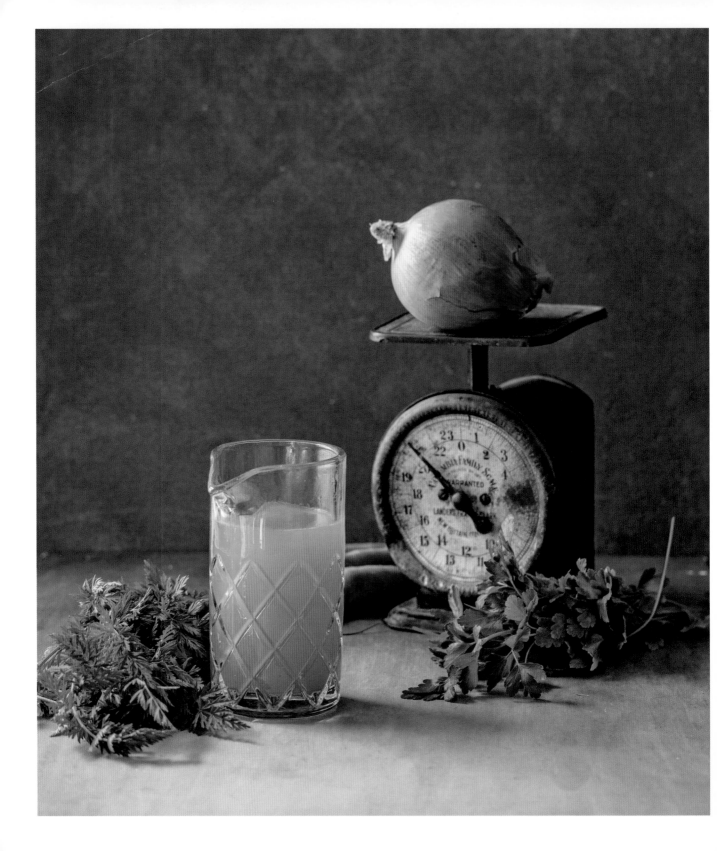

LOW-HISTAMINE CHICKEN BROTH

Broths are really worth making when you begin restricting your diet a little because they add a lot of flavor to other dishes, as well as nutrients and antioxidants to help soothe gut inflammation. They also add a shot of antihistamine power thanks to the herbs and spices. This chicken broth contains a lot of antihistamine allies. The thyme, onion, turmeric, garlic, kale, parsley and rosemary will all work in your favor as you enjoy consuming them. Omit the chicken to make it vegetarian or replace it with any meat for other options. Your dishes will sizzle with flavor.

MAKES ABOUT 12 CUPS (2.9 L)

1 tbsp (15 ml) olive oil

1 large onion, finely chopped

4 cloves garlic, finely chopped

4 medium carrots, finely chopped

4 large ribs celery, finely chopped

1 tsp sea salt, divided

9 to 10 cups (2.2 to 2.4 L) filtered water

1 cup (67 g) coarsely chopped kale, collards or Swiss chard

½ cup (30 g) coarsely chopped fresh parsley

3 or 4 sprigs fresh thyme

2 sprigs fresh rosemary

2 dried bay leaves

1 tsp turmeric

1 organic chicken carcass

Set the Instant Pot to the Sauté setting. Once the Instant Pot is hot, add the oil, onion, garlic, carrots, celery and ½ teaspoon of the salt. Sauté for about 5 minutes, or until the vegetables are softened and slightly browned, stirring frequently.

Add the water, kale, parsley, thyme, rosemary, bay leaves, turmeric and remaining ½ teaspoon salt. Add the chicken carcass to the mixture.

Close the lid of the Instant Pot and pressure-cook at high pressure for 120 minutes, then do a 15-minute natural release. After 15 minutes, turn the venting knob to the venting position to release the remaining pressure. Open the lid carefully and strain out the veggies.

Transfer the broth to silicone molds or freezer-safe Mason jars and store them in the freezer for later use.

KALE PESTO

Pesto is incredibly versatile and popular in my home. I find that having some on hand is incredibly useful when quick food preparation is necessary. It also adds a wonderful burst of flavor to any dish that needs perking up. If you are having trouble tolerating nuts, try removing them—you will still love the flavor!

MAKES APPROXIMATELY 1 CUP (252 G)

4 cups (268 g) packed torn kale leaves, stems removed

1 cup (24 g) packed fresh basil leaves

½ tsp sea salt

¾ cup (180 ml) extra-virgin olive oil

¼ cup (43 g) toasted almonds

1 clove garlic, coarsely chopped

Place the kale, basil, salt, oil, almonds and garlic in a food processor and blend on high until the desired consistency is reached. Add more oil if you prefer a thinner pesto. Freeze the leftover pesto in silicone ice cube trays and store them in silicone bags for up to 6 months.

PHASE 3: To make this recipe phase 3 compliant, omit the almonds.

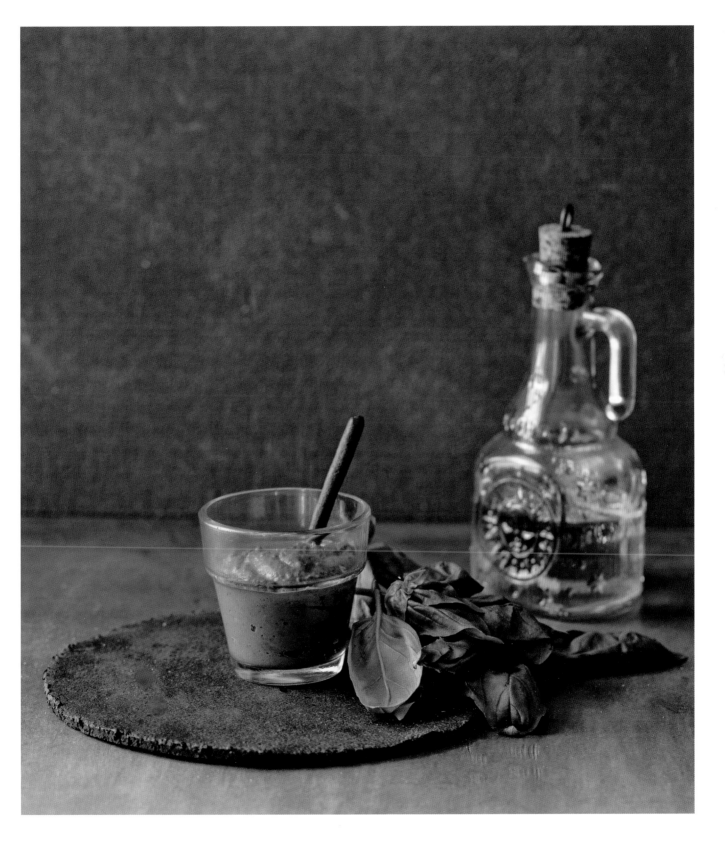

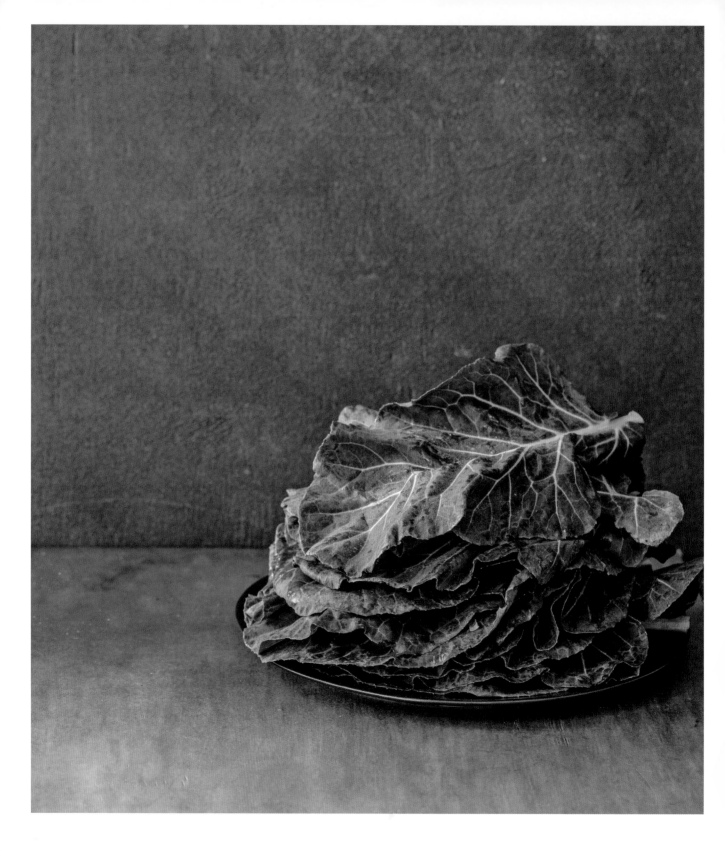

BLANCHED COLLARD GREEN WRAPS

Collard greens are mineral-rich and anti-inflammatory, but they also allow you to create a sandwich-like dish without any gluten. Use these in Kale and Onion Chicken Patty Wraps (page 107), Sweet and Savory Chicken Salad Wraps (page 108) and Chicken and Pesto Collard Wraps (page 111).

YIELD VARIES

Collard greens, as needed

Boil the collard greens for 2½ minutes, then transfer them directly to a bowl of ice water. Store the collard greens in the refrigerator for up to 3 days in a bag or sealed container.

TIGERNUT BUTTER

The tigernut, or chufa nut, is a chickpea-size superfood that has been used for centuries in Africa and is growing in popularity in the United States. Tigernuts are special because they are high in a type of resistance starch that can help with weight loss, boost digestive health and help prevent inflammatory bowel diseases. They are rich in iron, zinc, copper, magnesium and protein. Despite their name, they aren't nuts, so they're safe for this diet. However, they do have a sweet, nutty flavor to satisfy a nut craving. This nut butter can be converted into an antihistamine and low-carb butter by simply changing up the maple syrup for stevia.

MAKES 1 CUP (180 G)

1 cup (150 g) tigernuts or 1 cup (125 g) tigernut flour (page 67)

¼ to ½ cup (60 to 120 ml) extra-virgin olive oil

1 tsp preservative-free vanilla extract

1 tbsp (15 ml) maple syrup or local honey (optional) or 5 drops stevia (for low-carb; optional)

Pinch of sea salt

Place the tigernuts, oil, vanilla, maple syrup (if using) and salt in a blender and blend until smooth.

NOTE: Using tigernut flour is the easiest way to make this recipe and can be purchased on Amazon.

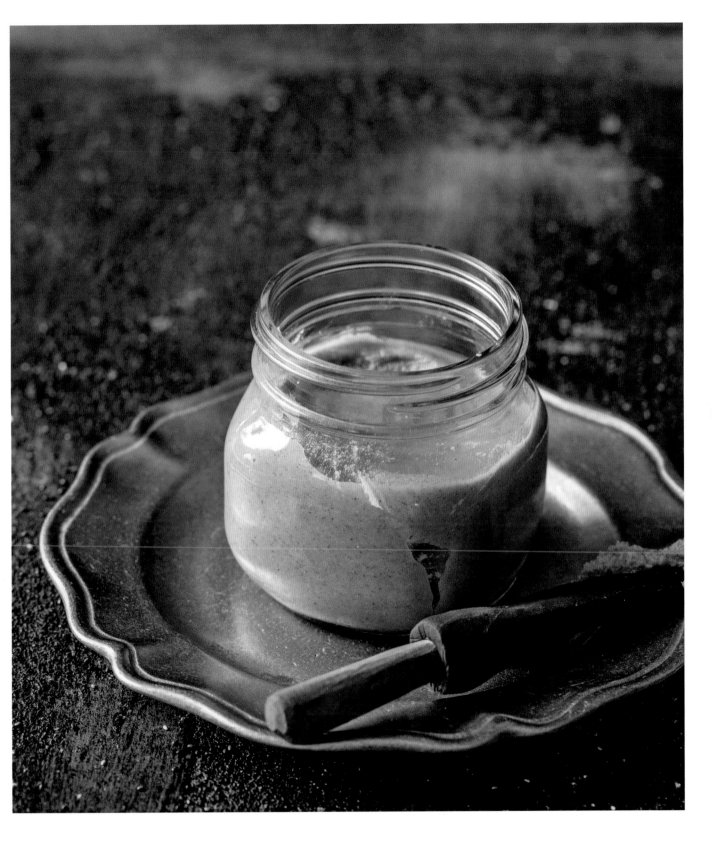

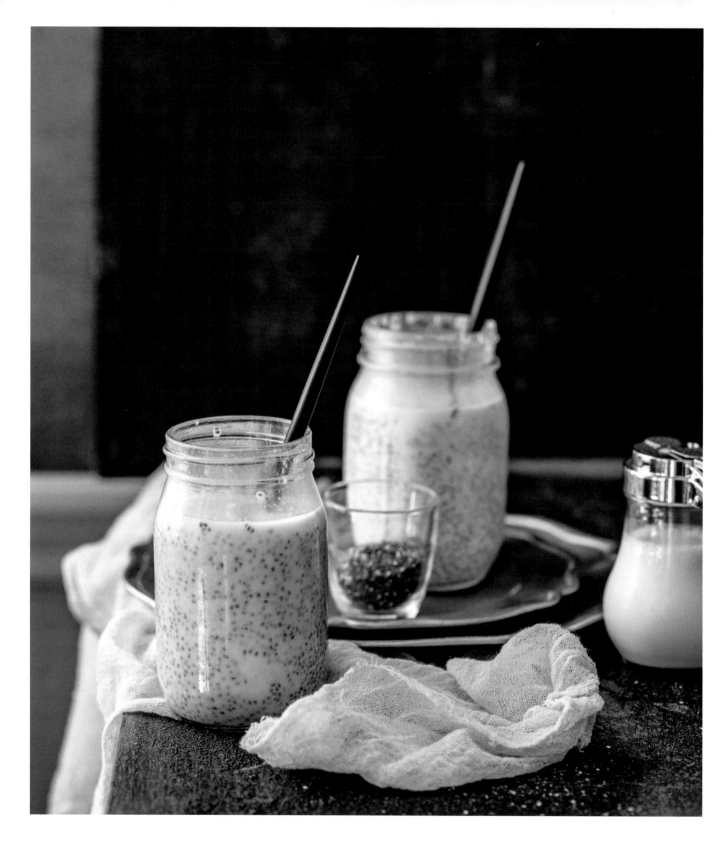

CHIA SEED PUDDING

Chia seeds have such a wide range of properties you can benefit from. These nutrient- and fiber-rich seeds create a gelatin-like substance in the gut that can act as a prebiotic, supporting the growth of probiotic bacteria. They help lower inflammation, too, as well as help you maintain steady energy levels. You can prepare this pudding in just a couple of minutes.

MAKES 1 SERVING

¼ cup (60 ml) canned coconut milk

¾ cup (180 ml) almond milk or coconut milk from a carton

¼ cup (41 g) chia seeds

1 tbsp (15 ml) maple syrup

1 tsp preservative-free vanilla extract

Place the coconut milk, almond milk, chia seeds, maple syrup and vanilla in a Mason jar and shake. Place the Mason jar in the refrigerator for at least 4 hours or overnight.

PHASE 3: Remove the almond milk and use 1 cup (240 ml) coconut milk if almonds are not tolerated.

BLUEBERRY JELLY

This is something you can make and freeze into silicone trays and use as you need. One frozen cube or 2 tablespoons (40 g) fresh is all that is needed for each serving of "PB and J" Chia Pudding (page 87).

MAKES ABOUT ¾ CUP (240 G)

1½ cups (220 g) fresh or thawed frozen blueberries

1 tbsp (15 ml) maple syrup or local honey

2 tsp (6 g) chia seeds

In a small pot over medium heat, combine the blueberries and maple syrup. Cook, stirring frequently, until the blueberries are cooked down, 5 to 10 minutes. Turn off the heat and stir in the chia seeds. Once the jelly is cool, it is ready to be served.

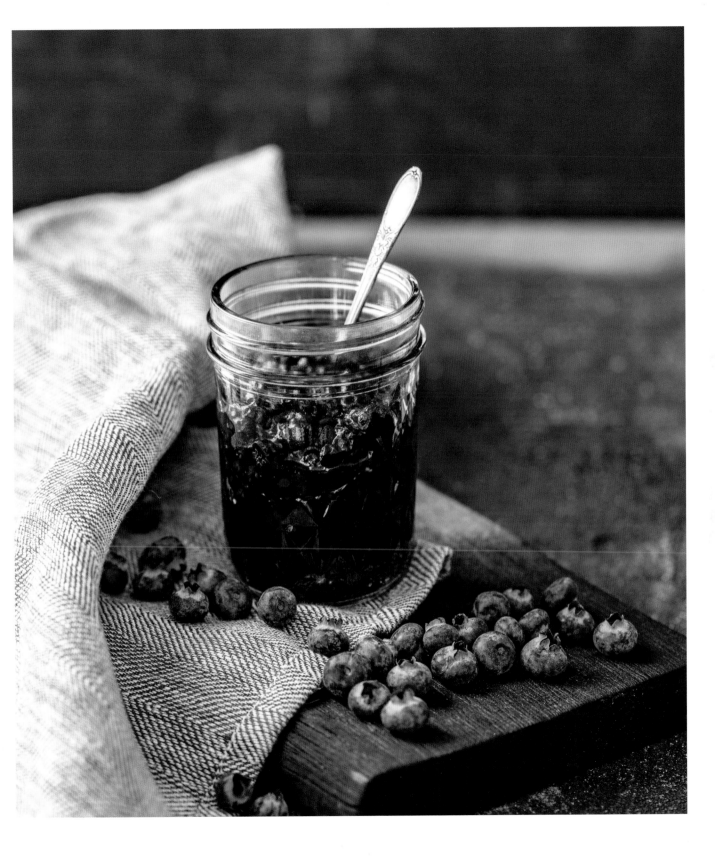

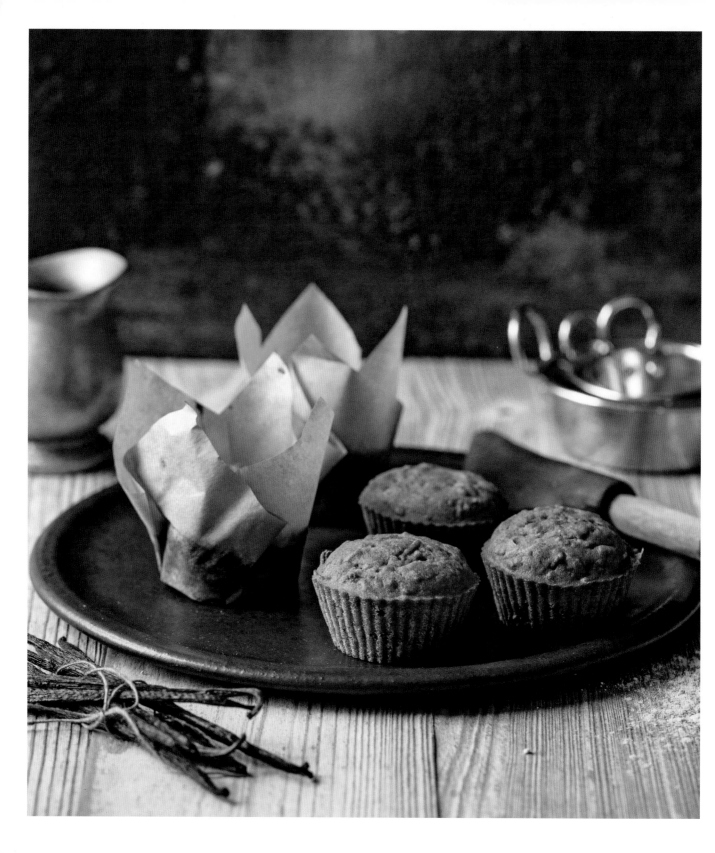

BREAKFAST

A healthy, low-histamine breakfast is important to set you up for a symptom-free day and help you resist nonprotocol foods all day long. I love having a premade breakfast, such as a chia pudding, in the refrigerator when I wake up—especially during the week, when I need to fly out the door with minimal fuss and food prep. This section includes cooked breakfasts and simple, quick options as well as my personal favorites for healthy, low-histamine morning meals.

APPLE AND CARROT MUFFINS

I always feel like I'm spoiling myself when I make this recipe, but this is one of the healthiest muffin recipes I have ever created thanks to healthy oils and added fiber from the apple and carrots.

MAKES 12 MUFFINS

3 large pasture-raised eggs

½ cup (72 g) maple or coconut sugar

½ cup (120 ml) coconut or almond milk

¼ cup (58 g) coconut oil, melted, or ¼ cup (60 ml) extra-light olive oil

2 tsp (10 ml) preservative-free vanilla extract

1 cup (125 g) tigernut flour (page 67)

½ cup (63 g) tapioca flour (page 66)

1 tsp baking soda

Pinch of sea salt

1 cup (120 g) peeled shredded apple

½ cup (25 g) shredded carrots

Preheat the oven to 350°F (177°C) and line a 12-well muffin pan with unbleached muffin liners.

In a large bowl, beat the eggs and add the sugar, coconut milk, oil and vanilla. Blend the mixture with a hand mixer until smooth.

In a small bowl, mix together the tigernut flour, tapioca flour, baking soda and salt.

Add the flour mixture to the egg mixture and mix until the two are blended together, being careful not to overmix. Fold in the apple and carrots.

Pour the batter into the muffin pan and bake for 20 to 22 minutes, until a toothpick inserted into the center of a muffin comes out clean. Let the muffins cool before serving.

APPLE BREAD

Missing doughy textures and essentially anything that contains gluten is absolutely normal when you cut out gluten. However, there are many ways to make an alternative that beats regular bread, in my mind. This bread's star ingredient—apples—contain quercetin, which keeps histamine at bay.

MAKES 12 SERVINGS

APPLE MIXTURE

1 tbsp (14 g) coconut oil

1 large Gala or Fuji apple, peeled and thinly sliced

2 tbsp (30 ml) maple syrup

1 tbsp (9 g) maple sugar

BREAD MIXTURE

3 large pasture-raised eggs

½ cup (123 g) applesauce

½ cup (120 ml) maple syrup

½ cup (120 ml) coconut or almond milk

2 tbsp (28 g) coconut oil, melted

2 tsp (10 ml) preservative-free vanilla extract

1 cup (96 g) almond flour (page 67)

½ cup (63 g) tapioca flour (page 66)

1 tsp baking soda

Pinch of sea salt

Preheat the oven to 350°F (177°C). Line a 9 x 5-inch (23 x 13-cm) bread pan with parchment paper.

To make the apple mixture, melt the coconut oil in a medium skillet over medium heat and add the apple. Add the maple syrup and maple sugar. Cook, stirring frequently, until the apples start to soften, about 7 minutes.

While the apples are cooking, make the bread mixture. In a large bowl, mix together the eggs, applesauce, maple syrup, coconut milk, oil and vanilla. In a medium bowl, combine the almond flour, tapioca flour, baking soda and salt. Add the flour mixture to the egg mixture and mix with a hand mixer until fully combined.

Pour half of the bread mixture into the prepared bread pan. Place half of the apple mixture on the bread mixture layer. Pour the rest of the bread mixture over the apple layer and make a second layer with the remaining apple mixture on the top.

Bake the bread for about 40 minutes, or until a toothpick inserted into the center comes out clean. Let the bread cool before serving.

PHASE 3: Omit the almond flour and use 1 cup (122 g) of cassava flour and ½ cup (63 g) of tapioca flour.

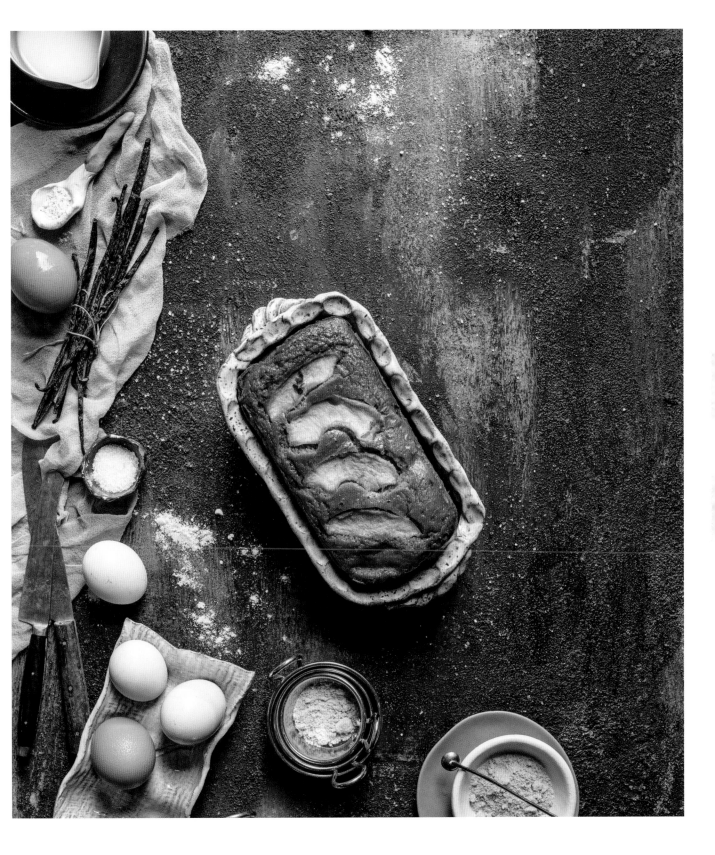

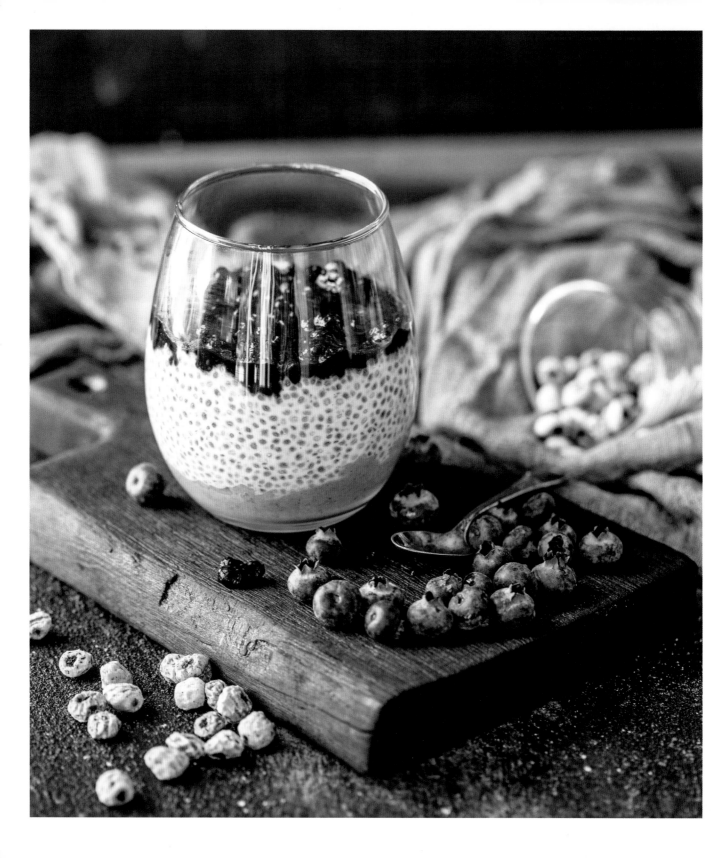

⅁DDING

...ed diet doesn't have to be boring or bland
...ely well, and the two are surprisingly light
...s layered on top of this pudding, there's
but don't forget to serve yourself some

...yer the Tigernut Butter on the bottom and Blueberry
...e Chia Seed Pudding and serve.

SPICED-UP EGGS OVER GREENS

Most people don't include many vegetables in their breakfast recipes, but consuming a portion or two of greens in your first meal of the day can help boost brain health and performance, as well as allow for more variety later. Cumin seeds are antihistamine, antioxidant and protect the mucosal lining of your digestive system, making this breakfast both therapeutic and appetizing.

MAKES 1 SERVING

2 tbsp (30 ml) olive oil, or grass-fed butter, divided

3 leaves Swiss chard, coarsely chopped

2 large pasture-raised eggs

⅛ tsp ground cumin

⅛ tsp garlic powder

⅛ tsp onion powder

Sea salt, to taste

Heat 1 tablespoon (15 ml) of the olive oil in a medium skillet over medium-high heat. Add the Swiss chard and sauté until it is very wilted, about 10 minutes. Push the Swiss chard to one side of the skillet.

Heat the remaining 1 tablespoon (15 ml) of olive oil in the skillet and add the eggs. Cook the eggs on each side to the desired consistency.

Sprinkle the cumin, garlic powder, onion powder and salt over the eggs and serve on top of the Swiss chard.

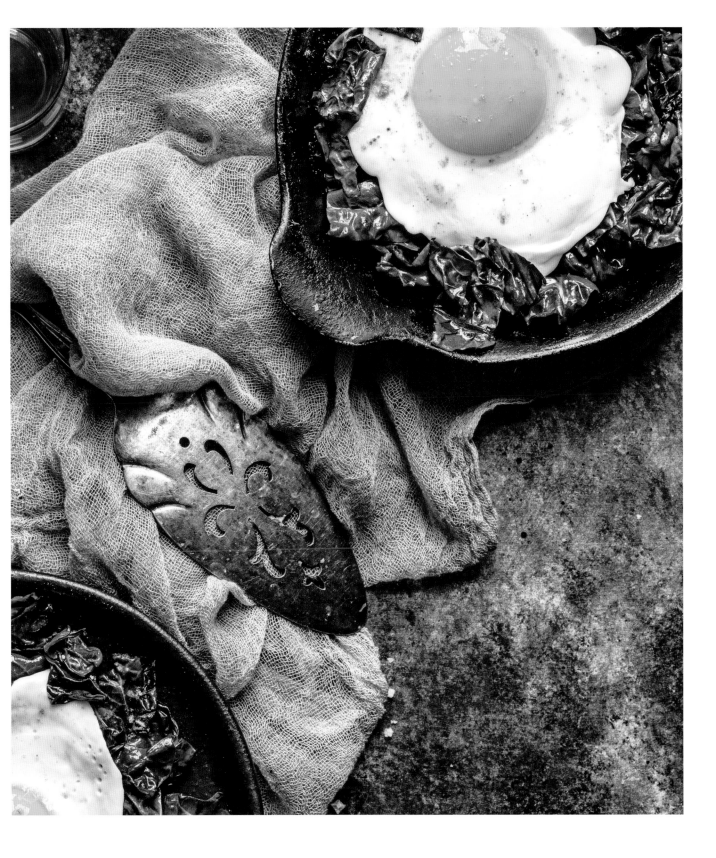

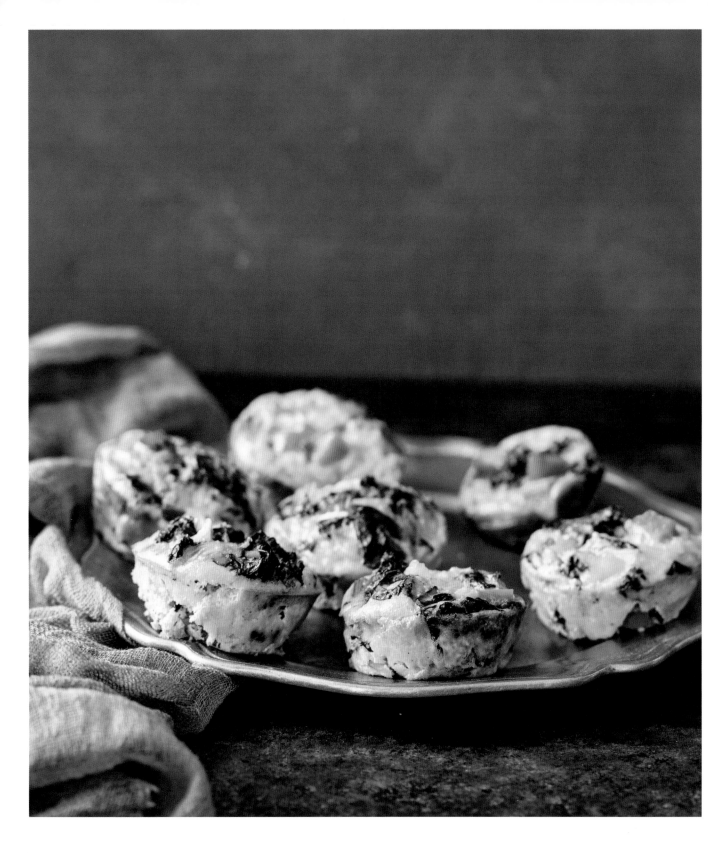

KALE AND SWEET POTATO EGG MUFFINS

If you're willing to make up a batch of these on Sunday, you could freeze them and be set for breakfast all week. The shape of these savory muffin cups makes them ideal for taking to work or school, and they will help you avoid unhealthy options that could tempt you to veer away from your antihistamine routine. The kale, sweet potato, shallots and garlic will all be working in your favor as you go about your morning.

MAKES 12 MUFFINS

2 tbsp (30 ml) olive oil

½ large sweet potato, peeled and cubed

4 cups (268 g) coarsely chopped kale

1 tsp sea salt, plus more to taste

3 shallots or ½ large Vidalia onion, finely chopped

10 large pasture-raised eggs

1 tsp garlic powder

1 tsp onion powder

Preheat the oven to 350°F (177°C). Line a muffin pan with baking cups.

Heat the olive oil in a medium skillet over medium-high heat. Add the sweet potato, kale and salt to taste and sauté for 5 minutes. Add the shallots and sauté for 5 more minutes. Transfer this mixture to a large glass or stainless steel bowl.

Add the eggs, 1 teaspoon salt, garlic powder and onion powder to the sweet potato mixture and mix well. Divide the mixture evenly among the muffin cups. Bake the muffins for 20 to 25 minutes, or until a fork inserted into the center comes out clean.

Freeze some of the muffins to eat later, if desired.

ASPARAGUS AND RED POTATO FRITTATA

Asparagus is loaded with nutrients and helps keep your blood sugar steady. Team it with the basil and onion, which both help prevent the symptoms of histamine intolerance as you go about your day, and you have the perfect breakfast for the whole family.

MAKES 6 TO 8 SERVINGS

2 tbsp (30 ml) extra-virgin olive oil

½ large Vidalia onion, finely chopped

8 to 10 asparagus spears, chopped into ½-inch (13-mm) pieces

1 red potato, peeled, shredded and squeezed of excess moisture

¾ tsp sea salt, divided

8 large pasture-raised eggs, beaten

¼ cup (10 g) coarsely chopped basil

2 tbsp (4 g) coarsely chopped chives

Preheat the oven to 400°F (204°C).

In a medium oven-safe skillet over medium-high heat, combine the oil, onion and asparagus and cook for 5 minutes. Add the potato and half the salt. Cook for 5 minutes.

Add the eggs, basil, chives and remaining salt to a medium bowl and mix well. Pour the egg mixture into the skillet and turn off the heat. Let the skillet sit on the hot burner until it is set and cooked through.

Transfer the skillet to the oven and bake until the frittata is puffed and cooked through, about 15 minutes. Remove the frittata from the oven and let it cool for 5 minutes before serving.

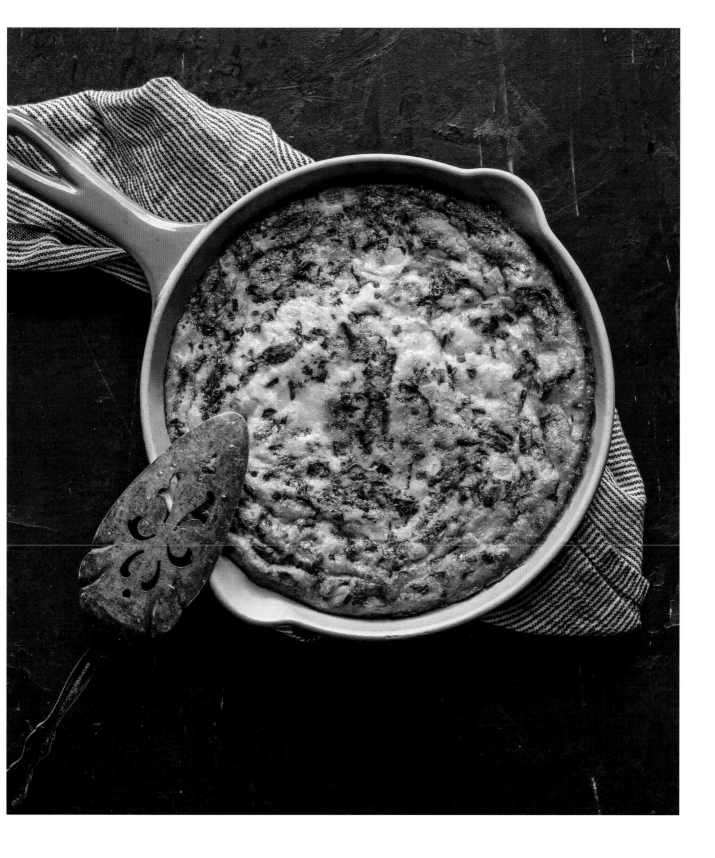

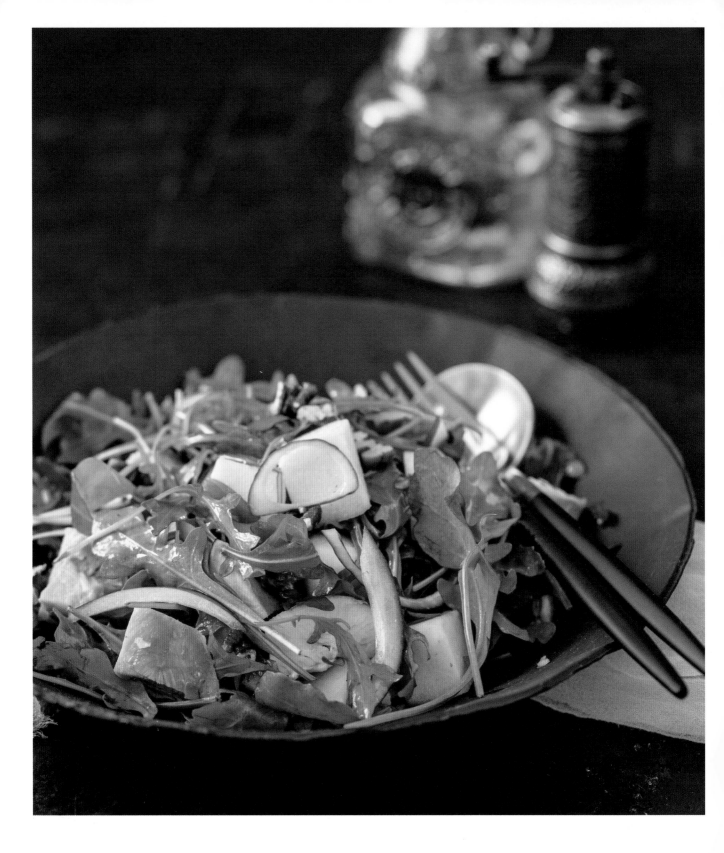

LUNCH

Lunch is an important meal to keep your energy steady later in the afternoon and prevent the temptation to snack on foods that aren't part of your elimination diet mid-afternoon. No matter if you would like a light lunch or something more elaborate, this section will have plenty of options for you. I have included as many options as possible that can be made ahead of time and frozen for easy use each day.

APPLE, PECAN AND CHICKEN ARUGULA SALAD

This fun salad is packed with antioxidant-rich pecans, which also help reduce inflammation and contain more than 19 vitamins and minerals. Apples and arugula both help diminish histamine levels in the body.

MAKES 1 SERVING

4 cups (80 g) arugula

1 small apple (any variety), peeled, cored and cubed

1 to 2 thin slices red onion

¼ cup (30 g) raw pecans, coarsely chopped

3 oz (84 g) cooked frozen chicken tenderloins (page 66) or cooked fresh chicken breast

Salad dressing of your choice (pages 170–171), to taste

Place the arugula, apple, onion, pecans and chicken in a medium bowl. Toss the salad with the salad dressing and serve.

PHASE 3: Remove the pecans if you do not tolerate them.

CHICKEN SAUSAGE, KALE AND SWEET POTATO SOUP

Perfect for the colder months, this soup combines mild, rich flavors from the Italian sausage, with antihistamine and high-quercetin ingredients to soothe the body. Most people tolerate chicken sausage well because it is not a dried sausage, which contains higher histamine levels. If you find you cannot tolerate chicken sausage, you can substitute it with ground chicken.

MAKES 6 TO 8 SERVINGS

2 tbsp (30 ml) extra-virgin olive oil

1 lb (450 g) organic, nitrate-free mild Italian chicken sausage or ground organic chicken, rolled into small balls

1 medium Vidalia onion, coarsely chopped

2 cloves garlic, minced

1 large sweet potato, peeled and cubed

2 large carrots, cut into ¼-inch (6-mm)-thick pieces

2 cups (180 g) coarsely chopped green cabbage

1 medium bunch Tuscan kale, stems removed, coarsely chopped

1½ tsp (2 g) Italian seasoning

6 cups (1.4 L) Low-Histamine Chicken Broth (page 71)

Sea salt and pepper, to taste

Heat the oil in a large stockpot over medium heat. Add the chicken sausage balls and onion and sauté until the sausage is thoroughly cooked through, about 10 minutes.

Add the garlic, sweet potato, carrots, cabbage, kale and Italian seasoning and cook for 3 to 5 minutes.

Add the broth and bring the mixture to a simmer. Simmer for 15 to 20 minutes, or until the sweet potato is tender.

Add the salt and pepper, if needed. (I do not add any more if using the chicken sausage but I do if using ground chicken.)

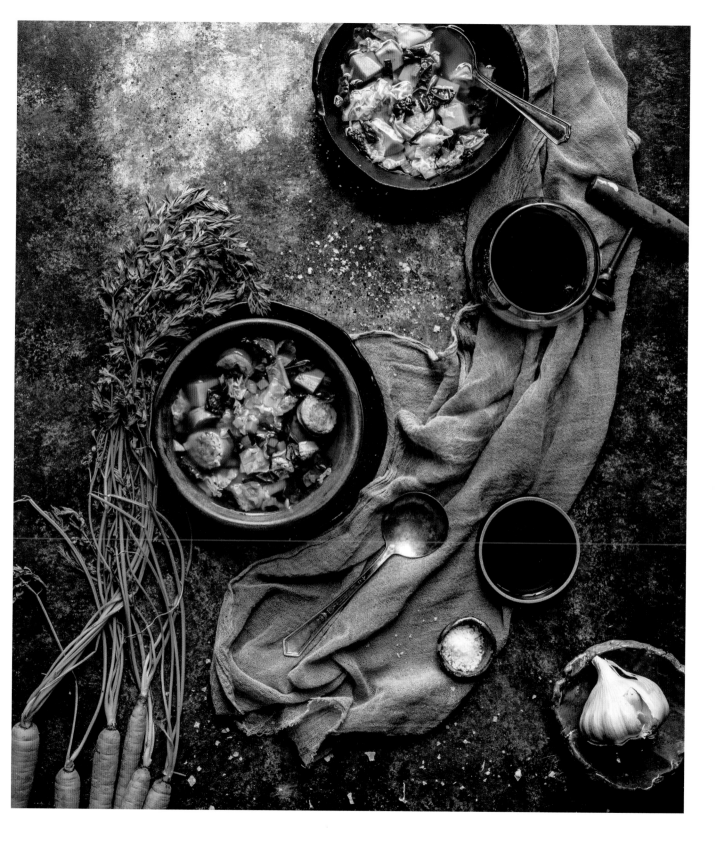

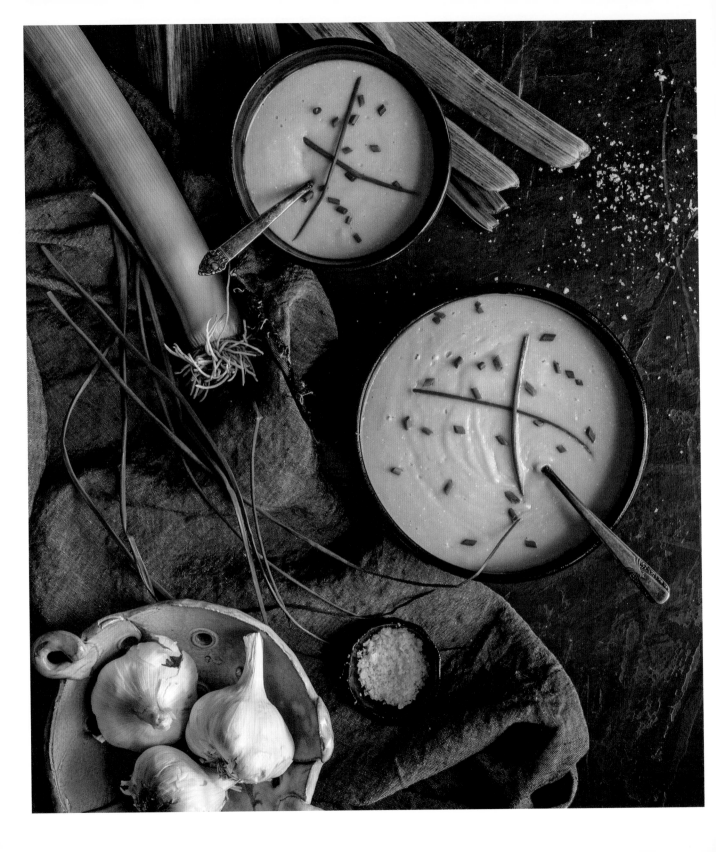

ARTICHOKE SOUP

Liquids are inherently digestible, making this soup healthy and light on your digestion. It contains artichokes, which are rich in luteolin, an antioxidant that reduces mast cell activation. Artichokes are also full of fiber, protein and prebiotic power, enabling this soup to pack an even greater nutritional punch.

MAKES 6 TO 8 SERVINGS

2 tbsp (28 g) grass-fed butter

2 large leeks, white parts only, thinly sliced

2 medium russet or red potatoes, peeled and coarsely chopped

2 cloves garlic, minced

1 (12-oz [336-g]) package frozen artichoke hearts, thawed

4 cups (960 ml) Low-Histamine Chicken or Vegetable Broth (page 71)

1 tsp sea salt

¾ cup (180 ml) canned coconut cream

Coarsely chopped chives, for garnish

Set the Instant Pot to the Sauté setting. Add the butter to the pot and allow it to melt, then add the leeks and potatoes. Stir and cook for 5 minutes, adding the garlic during the final minute.

Add the artichokes, broth and salt and turn off the Instant Pot. Place the lid on the Instant Pot and choose the Soup setting. Adjust the pressure to high and use the default cook time set by the Instant Pot.

Once the timer is done, use the quick-release option. Remove the lid and stir in the coconut cream, then allow the mixture to cool.

Once the mixture has cooled, transfer it to a blender and puree (or use an immersion blender to puree the soup).

If needed, transfer the soup back to the Instant Pot to reheat it. Or you can transfer the soup to freezer-safe Mason jars (leaving 1 inch [2.5 cm] of space at the top) and freeze it for your lunches for the week. Sprinkle with chives before serving.

This soup can also be made on the stove in a large stockpot by increasing the cooking time to 20 minutes.

ROSEMARY AND GARLIC LAMB BURGERS

This recipe is a family favorite. As you know, garlic is both antihistamine and anti-inflammatory. Rosemary, which enhances digestion and protects the brain, also pairs very nicely with lamb.

MAKES 4 SERVINGS

1 lb (450 g) organic ground lamb

2 tbsp (4 g) coarsely chopped fresh rosemary

2 to 3 cloves garlic, minced

8 leaves butter or iceberg lettuce

Combine the lamb, rosemary and garlic in a medium bowl and mix well. Form the lamb mixture into 4 patties and either freeze them in single-serving portions or cook them in a medium skillet over medium-high heat for 3 to 5 minutes per side and serve them fresh, wrapping each burger in 2 lettuce leaves as a bun.

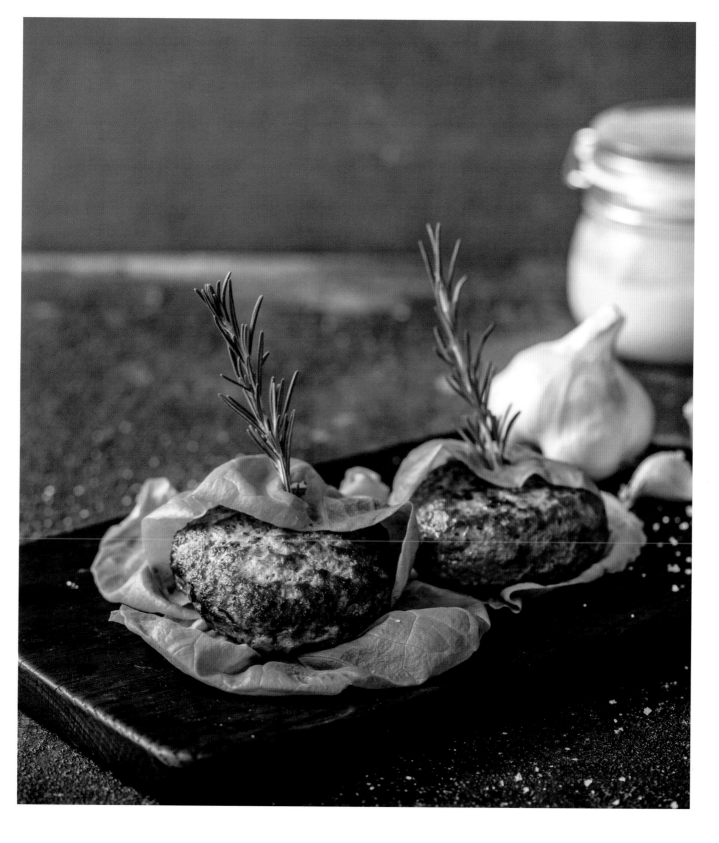

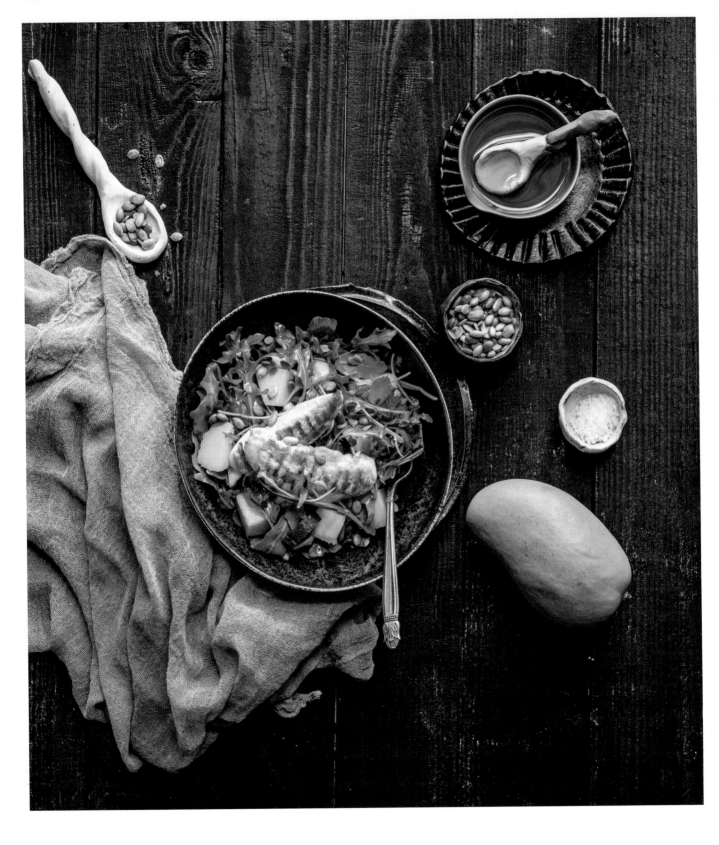

CHICKEN AND MANGO SALAD

Mango is another histamine-fighting fruit that goes unexpectedly well with chicken. The freshness of the cucumbers makes this a very nice, light meal that's perfect for summer.

MAKES 1 SERVING

3 oz (84 g) frozen organic chicken tenderloin (page 66), thawed, or fresh chicken breast

Sea salt

2 cups (40 g) arugula

½ cup (83 g) cubed fresh mango

¼ cup (30 g) roasted pumpkin seeds

½ medium cucumber, coarsely chopped

Ginger Dressing (page 171), to taste

Sprinkle the chicken with the salt. Place the chicken in a medium skillet over medium-high heat and cook until it is completely cooked through, 3 to 5 minutes on each side.

In a medium bowl, combine the arugula, mango, pumpkin seeds and cucumber. Top the salad with the chicken and drizzle it with the dressing.

CHICKEN AND SAGE "NOODLE" SOUP

Who said noodle soup couldn't be gluten-free? Spaghetti squash is another antihistamine food and creates an authentic-feeling texture to this hearty soup.

MAKES 6 TO 8 SERVINGS

1 large spaghetti squash, cut in half vertically

6 cups (1.4 L) water, divided

3 tbsp (42 g) butter or 3 tbsp (45 ml) extra-virgin olive oil

1 cup (150 g) coarsely chopped onion

3 tbsp (27 g) arrowroot powder

1 cup (128 g) coarsely chopped carrots

1 cup (100 g) coarsely chopped celery

4 cups (960 ml) Low-Histamine Chicken Broth (page 71), divided

2 tbsp (4 g) coarsely chopped fresh sage

2 tbsp (4 g) coarsely chopped fresh parsley

1½ lb (675 g) boneless, skinless organic chicken breast, cubed

Sea salt, as needed

Set the squash on a trivet in the Instant Pot and add 2 cups (480 ml) of the water. Set the Instant Pot on the Manual setting and set the time for 7 minutes, making sure the valve is closed.

When the timer is done, turn the valve for a quick release and turn off the Instant Pot. Remove the squash and set it on a worksurface. Scrape out the "noodles" with a fork. Pour out the liquid remaining in the bottom of the insert and return the insert to the Instant Pot.

Set the Instant Pot to the Sauté setting. Melt the butter in the Instant Pot. Add the onion and cook until translucent, about 5 minutes, then add the arrowroot powder and stir to combine. Add the carrots, celery and 1 cup (240 ml) of the broth and cook until the vegetables are tender, about 3 minutes. Stir in the sage and parsley and cook until fragrant, about 1 minute.

Season the chicken with the salt. Add the chicken, remaining 3 cups (720 ml) of broth and 4 cups (960 ml) of water to the Instant Pot. Turn off the Instant Pot and turn it to the Soup setting. Adjust the pressure to high and set the time for 10 minutes.

When the timer goes off, do a quick release and open the lid. Turn the setting back to Sauté and add the spaghetti squash "noodles." Stir to combine and cook, uncovered, for about 5 minutes.

This recipe can be done in a large stockpot as well. Use the exact same directions but adjust the cook time to 15 to 20 minutes.

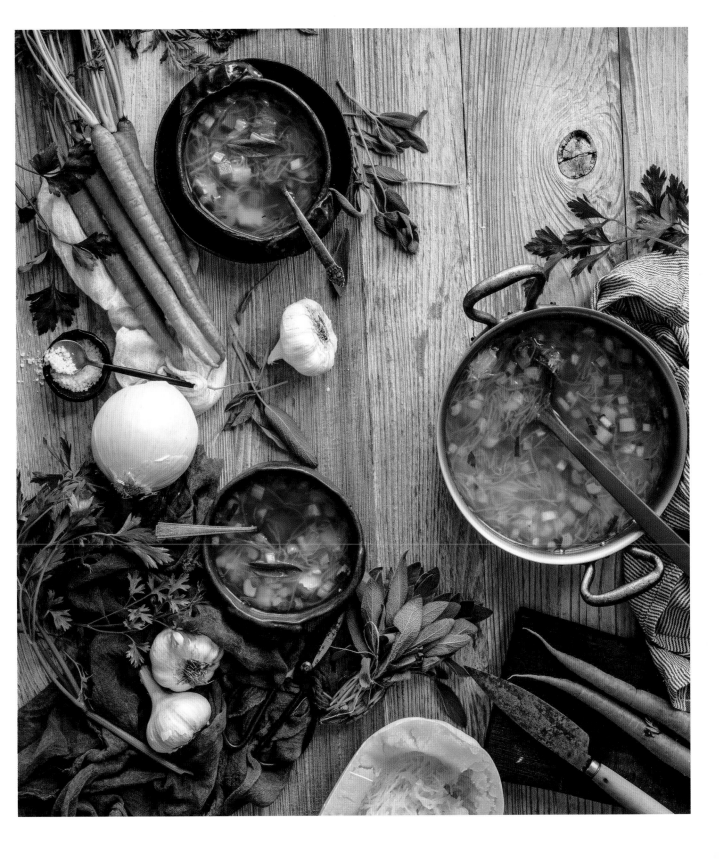

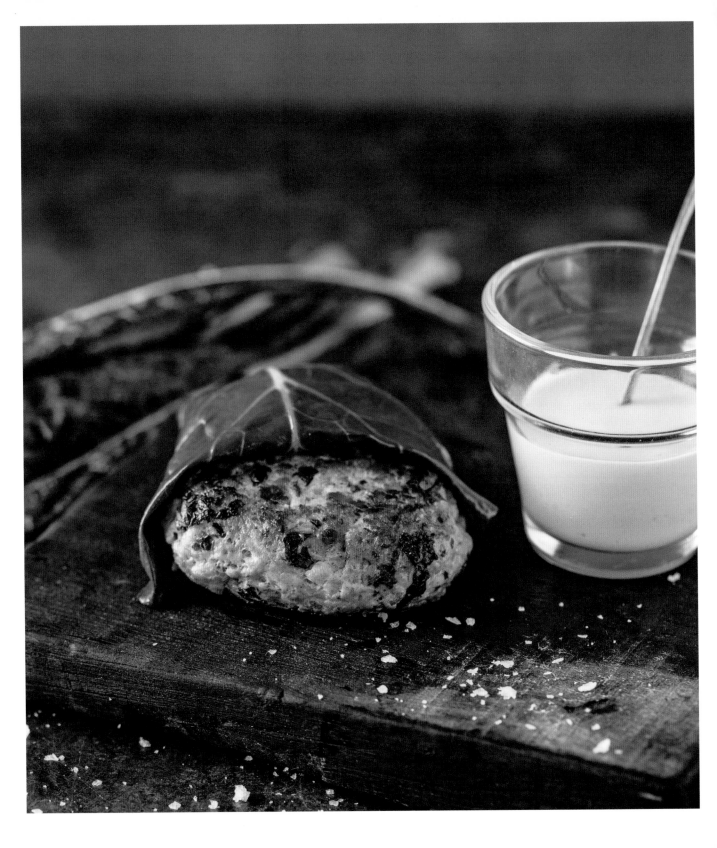

KALE AND ONION CHICKEN PATTY WRAPS

These patty wraps are wonderfully quick and easy to make and can be frozen ahead of time to ensure you always have something delicious on hand for any occasion.

MAKES 4 SERVINGS

1 lb (450 g) ground organic chicken

2 cups (134 g) finely chopped kale

½ medium onion, finely chopped

1 tsp sea salt

4 Blanched Collard Green Wraps (page 75)

Lower-Histamine Mayonnaise (page 68)

Butter lettuce leaves, as needed

In a large bowl, combine the chicken, kale, onion and salt. Form this mixture into 4 patties and either freeze them immediately to use later or cook them in a medium skillet over medium-high heat for 3 to 5 minutes on each side and serve immediately.

Serve each patty on a collard green wrap with the mayonnaise and lettuce.

SWEET AND SAVORY CHICKEN SALAD WRAPS

With a sweet twist, these chicken wraps provide high-quercetin and antihistamine ingredients, while being just filling enough to keep you going all afternoon.

MAKES 4 SERVINGS

1 (3- to 4-lb [1.4- to 1.8-kg]) organic chicken

1 cup (240 ml) water

1 cup (220 g) Lower-Histamine Mayonnaise (page 68)

½ small onion, grated

½ cup (25 g) matchstick or grated carrots

Sea salt and pepper, to taste

4 Blanched Collard Green Wraps (page 75) or NUCO Coconut Wraps (page 177)

Place the chicken on a trivet in the Instant Pot and add the water to the bottom of the pot. Push the Poultry button and then adjust the Instant Pot to its maximum temperature. Manually increase the time to 35 minutes and make sure the valve is closed.

Once the chicken is done cooking, allow it to cool, and remove all the meat from the bones. Place the chicken in a medium bowl and shred it with two forks or your hands.

In another medium bowl, combine the shredded chicken, mayonnaise, onion, carrots, salt and pepper. Serve the chicken salad in the collard green wraps.

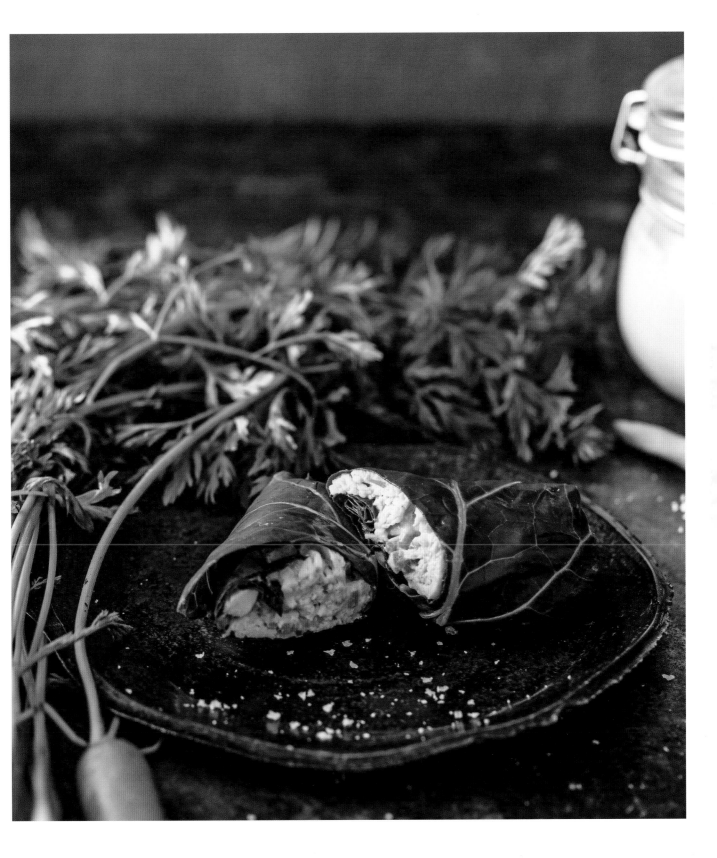

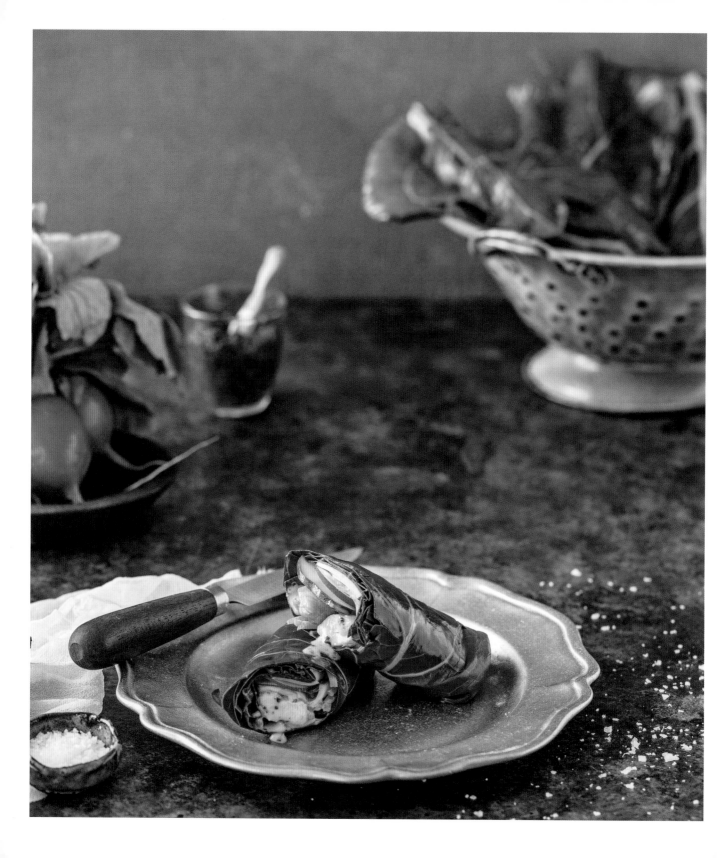

CHICKEN AND PESTO COLLARD WRAPS

I have found that most guests enjoy pesto, but this wrap has a fresh, crunchy touch that makes it perfect for lunchtime or an active day.

MAKES 1 SERVING

2 to 3 frozen organic chicken tenderloins, thawed (page 66)

Extra-virgin olive oil, as needed

Sea salt, as needed

1 tsp Lower-Histamine Mayonnaise (page 68)

1 tsp Kale Pesto (page 72)

1 Blanched Collard Green Wrap (page 75)

Cucumber slices, matchstick carrots, radish slices or any other veggies of choice

Coat the chicken with the oil on both sides and sprinkle it with the salt on both sides. Cook the chicken in a medium skillet or on a medium grill pan over medium-high heat until it is cooked through, 3 to 5 minutes.

Meanwhile, spread the mayo and pesto on the collard wrap.

Once the chicken is done, place it on the collard wrap near the middle and top it with the veggies of your choice. Wrap the collard leaf as you would a burrito. Cut in half and serve.

THYME AND OREGANO TURKEY BURGERS

Turkey always reminds me of the holiday season, but these turkey patties can be made any time of the year because they're so easy to throw together: wrap in butter lettuce leaves, smear with mayo and serve to the whole family.

MAKES 4 SERVINGS

1 lb (450 g) ground organic turkey

1 tbsp (2 g) finely chopped fresh thyme

1 tbsp (2 g) finely chopped fresh oregano

½ tsp sea salt

Butter lettuce leaves, as needed

Lower-Histamine Mayonnaise (page 68)

Combine the turkey, thyme, oregano and salt in a medium bowl and form the mixture into 4 patties. Cook the patties in a medium skillet over medium-high heat for 3 to 5 minutes on each side, or until the burgers are cooked through. (Alternatively, cook as many as you are serving and freeze the rest in individual servings to use later.)

Serve the burgers on the butter lettuce leaves with the mayonnaise and any other toppings you like.

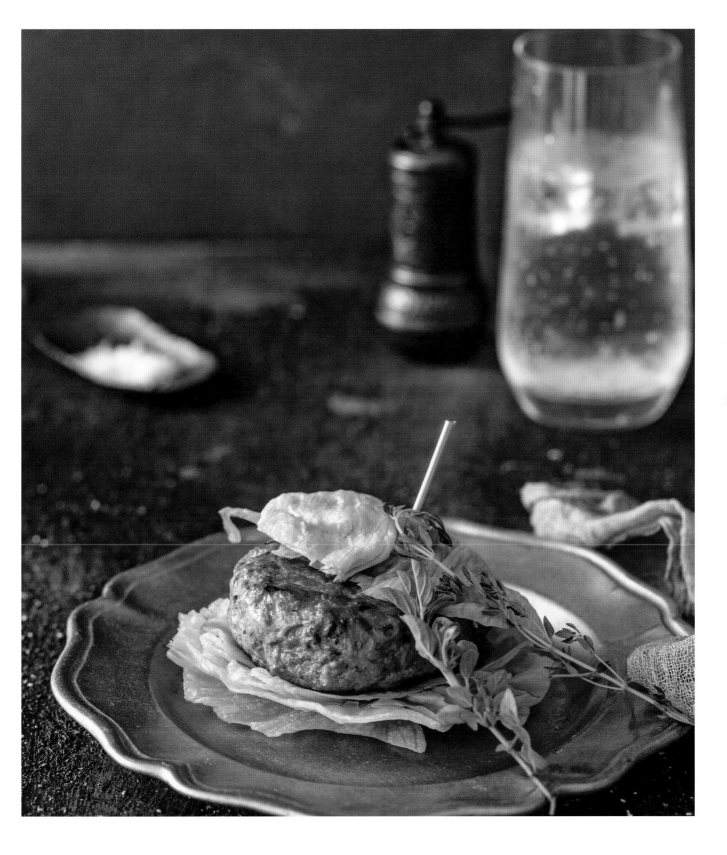

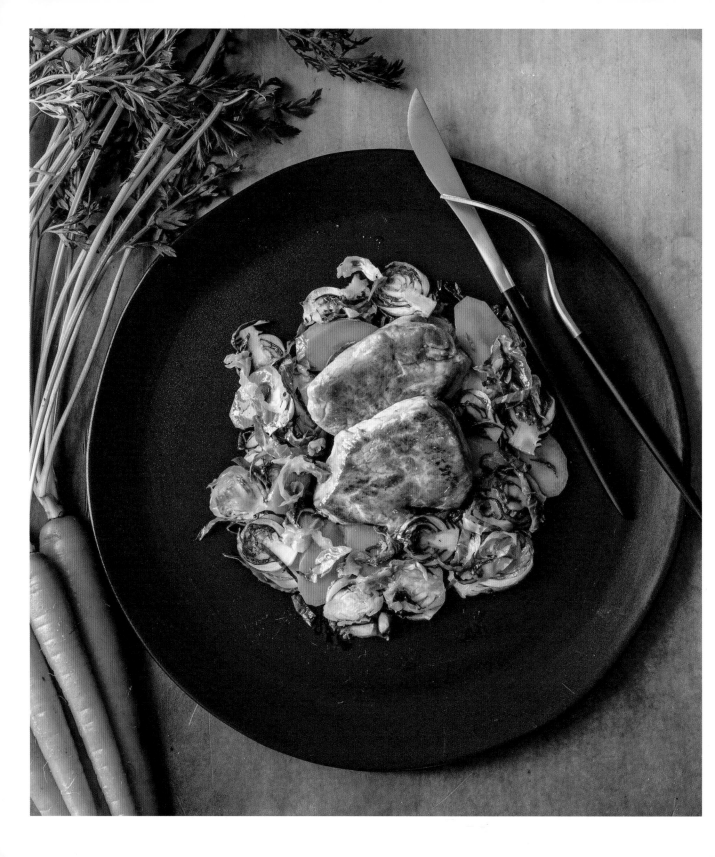

DINNER

Some find dinners daunting because they include the whole family. But that doesn't need to be the case, because here I offer you some hearty, healthy dinner recipes that are easy to make and don't have to be time-consuming to be delicious and well received. Make sure you add another side of veggies from the side dishes (pages 138–153) to each dinner that does not provide an adequate amount (see page 63) to give you the proper ratio of veggies to protein. This will be listed out for you in the meal plan on page 172.

PORK MEDALLIONS WITH SHAVED BRUSSELS AND CARROTS

Brussels sprouts are similar to cabbage in that they contain the healthy amino acid L-glutamine, which can aid in healing the gut. This filling combination of ingredients is perfect for the whole family, particularly during the colder months of the year.

MAKES 4 SERVINGS

4 tbsp (60 ml) extra-virgin olive oil, divided

1 (1½- to 2-lb [675- to 900-g]) organic pork tenderloin, cut into 1-inch (2.5-cm)-thick medallions

1 lb (450 g) Brussels sprouts, shaved in a food processor, divided

4 to 5 large carrots, cut into ¼-inch (6-mm)-thick slices

2 cloves garlic, coarsely chopped

½ cup (120 ml) coconut aminos

Heat a large cast-iron skillet over medium-high heat and add 2 tablespoons (30 ml) of the oil. Once the oil is hot, add the pork medallions to one side of the skillet and ½ pound (225 g) of the Brussels sprouts to the other side of the skillet. Cook for 3 to 5 minutes, then flip the pork medallions over and add the carrots to the Brussels sprouts and mix the two together. Add the remaining 2 tablespoons (30 ml) of oil at this point if needed. Cook 3 to 5 minutes, and when the pork is mostly cooked through, add the remaining ½ pound (225 g) of Brussels sprouts, the garlic and coconut aminos and mix everything together. Cook for 1 minute. Remove the skillet from the heat and serve.

HONEY–GARLIC CHICKEN

Garlic has been shown to inhibit histamine release from mast cells. It also fights inflammation and pathogens of various types and packs an antioxidant punch. Combine it with a soothing, anti-inflammatory honey sauce and some high-quality organic chicken, and you have a comforting, delicious, health-supporting meal!

MAKES 4 SERVINGS

SAUCE

3 tbsp (45 ml) local honey

1 tsp maple sugar

2 tbsp (30 ml) coconut aminos

3 tbsp (45 ml) Low-Histamine Chicken Broth (page 71)

CHICKEN

4 organic boneless, skinless chicken thighs

Sea salt and pepper, as needed

2 tbsp (28 g) coconut oil, divided

4 cloves garlic, minced

Coarsely chopped fresh parsley (optional)

To make the sauce, combine the honey, sugar, coconut aminos and broth in a small pot over high heat. Bring the sauce to a boil, then turn off the heat and set the sauce aside.

To make the chicken, place the chicken thighs on a paper towel and sprinkle the skin side with the salt and pepper.

Turn the Instant Pot to the Sauté setting and wait for it to say "Hot." Once the Instant Pot is hot, add 1 tablespoon (14 g) of the oil and the chicken thighs, skin side down. Brown the thighs for about 3 minutes and flip them over. Add additional salt and pepper and cook for 3 minutes, or until the thighs are browned.

Remove the chicken from the Instant Pot and set aside. Add the remaining 1 tablespoon (14 g) of oil and the garlic to the Instant Pot and cook for about 30 seconds. Transfer the chicken back to the pot and cover it with the sauce, mixing everything together so the garlic rises to the top. Put the lid on the Instant Pot and set it to Manual for 10 minutes.

Do a quick release when the timer goes off. When the valve drops, remove the cover carefully. Add the parsley, if using, to the chicken and serve immediately.

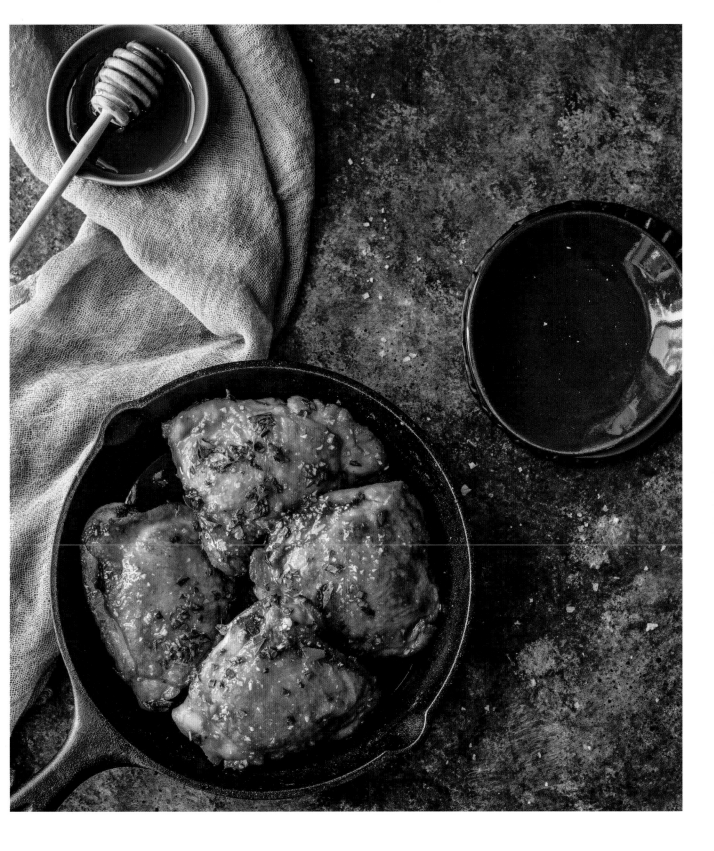

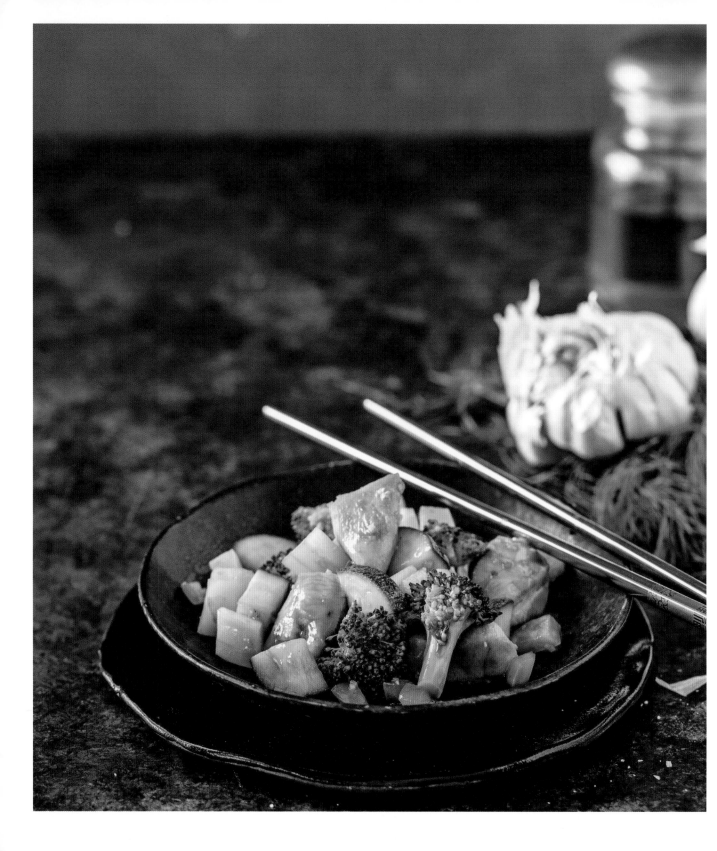

ANTIHISTAMINE CHICKEN STIR-FRY

This dish is a tasty way to add a good portion of vegetables to your day and benefit from the properties of the herbs and spices I have included. Fennel is high in quercetin, a great histamine blocker, and its flavor can instantly make any dish more interesting. Garlic helps keep bad bacteria at bay, supports the liver and contains plenty of antioxidants, as well as adds a lovely aromatic quality to this plate.

MAKES 6 SERVINGS

4 tbsp (60 ml) extra-virgin olive oil, divided

2 boneless, skinless organic chicken breasts, cut into bite-size pieces

1 medium Vidalia onion, chopped

1 large head fennel, chopped

4 cups (700 g) broccoli florets

1 medium zucchini, quartered and sliced to create half moons

6 tbsp (90 ml) coconut aminos, divided

1½ tbsp (11 g) minced ginger

3 cloves garlic, minced

Sea salt, to taste

Heat 2 tablespoons (30 ml) of the oil in a medium skillet over medium-high heat. Add the chicken and cook until it is cooked through, about 10 minutes. Set the chicken aside.

While the chicken is cooking, add the remaining 2 tablespoons (30 ml) of oil to a wok over medium-high heat. Add the onion and fennel and cook for about 10 minutes.

Add the broccoli, zucchini and 4 tablespoons (60 ml) of the coconut aminos to the wok and cook for 5 minutes. Add the ginger and garlic and cook for 5 minutes.

Stir the chicken and remaining 2 tablespoons (30 ml) of coconut aminos into the vegetables and cook for 1 minute. Season with salt.

INSTANT POT CHICKEN WITH GRAVY AND CAULIFLOWER MASH

The Instant Pot takes the long cooking time out of meals, which can decrease the histamine load and transform cooking into a delightfully easy experience. I have added thyme here for some added vitamin C and flavonoids to stabilize mast cells. The gravy adds a familiar, more sumptuous feel to this dish without adding any gluten.

MAKES 4 SERVINGS

CHICKEN

4 tbsp (60 ml) extra-virgin olive oil, divided

3 cloves garlic, minced

2 tsp (2 g) coarsely chopped fresh thyme

1 tsp sea salt

1 (4-lb [1.8-kg]) organic chicken

2 cups (480 ml) Low-Histamine Beef or Chicken Broth (page 71)

GRAVY

3 tbsp (42 g) grass-fed butter

3 tbsp (27 g) arrowroot powder

Sea salt and pepper, to taste

Cauliflower Mash (page 122)

To make the chicken, combine 2 tablespoons (30 ml) of the oil, garlic, thyme and salt in a small bowl and set aside. Press the Sauté button on the Instant Pot, so that it is on the Normal setting.

Add the remaining 2 tablespoons (30 ml) of oil to the pot, then add the chicken, breast side down, and brown for 4 minutes. While the breast side is browning, coat the bottom of the chicken with half of the oil mixture. Turn the chicken over using tongs and brown it on the bottom for 1 minute. While the bottom side is browning, coat the top of the chicken with the remaining oil mixture.

Remove the chicken from the pot with tongs and set it aside. Place a trivet in the bottom of the Instant Pot and add the broth. Place the chicken back in the Instant Pot on the trivet. Press the Cancel button and then the Poultry button. Then press Manual and increase to More. Adjust the time to 30 minutes, make sure the valve is sealed and cook the chicken. If the chicken is fewer than 4 pounds (1.8 kg), cook it for 25 minutes.

Once the timer goes off, allow the Instant Pot to depressurize naturally, about 15 minutes. Remove the chicken from the pot and set it aside. Reserve 2 cups (480 ml) of the cooking liquid from the pot and set it aside for the gravy. Reserve the rest of the liquid for the Cauliflower Mash (page 122).

To make the gravy, set the Instant Pot to Sauté. Add the butter and arrowroot powder and cook for 1 minute, whisking if needed to remove lumps. Slowly add the reserved 2 cups (480 ml) of cooking liquid while continuing to stir. Cook, stirring, until the gravy begins to thicken. Add the salt and pepper and serve with the chicken and Cauliflower Mash (page 122).

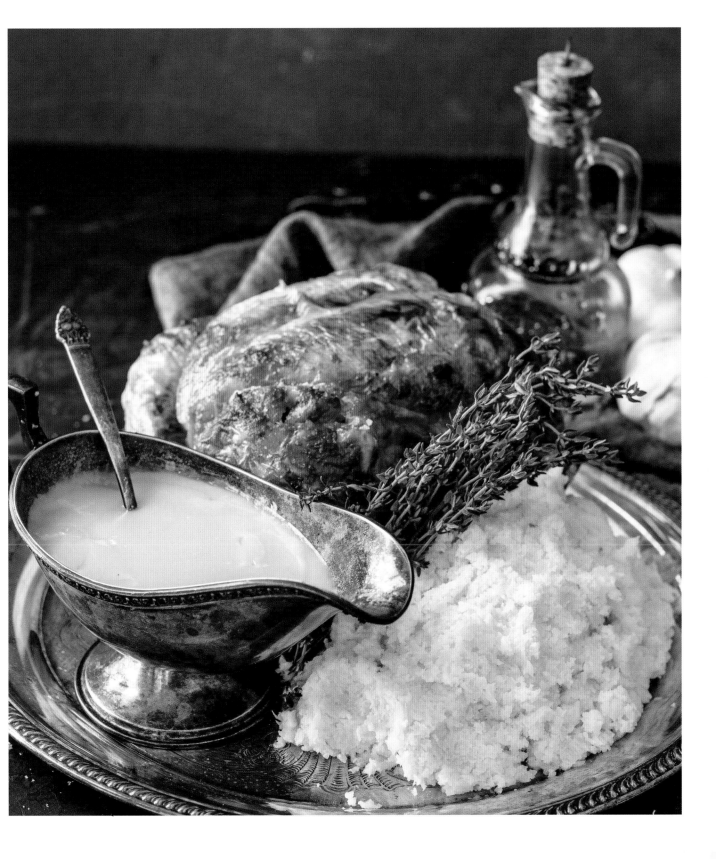

CAULIFLOWER MASH

Have you ever tried mash made from butternut squash or another type of squash? This side serves a similar function, but it is low-carb and high in choline, antioxidants and fiber, and it helps strengthen the immune system and promote detoxification. It also makes a wonderful base for savory and rich flavors.

MAKES 4 SERVINGS

1 large head organic cauliflower, chopped into florets

2 tbsp (28 g) grass-fed butter

¼ to ⅓ cup (60 to 80 ml) leftover liquid from Instant Pot Chicken (page 120)

½ tsp sea salt

Add the cauliflower to a large pot and cover the florets with water. Bring the water to a boil over medium-high heat and cook the cauliflower for 15 minutes. Drain the cauliflower and let it cool for about 10 minutes.

Place the cooled cauliflower, butter, half the broth and the salt in a food processor. Process on high speed until the cauliflower mixture is smooth and creamy, adding more broth as needed to reach the desired consistency.

SESAME-GINGER CHICKEN TACOS IN JICAMA SHELLS

Tacos are such a popular food, but consuming corn can be a bad idea because the protein present in corn can disrupt the gut lining and create problems in the digestive system. Most of the corn available to buy is also genetically modified. This taco recipe is corn-free and contains histamine intolerance–friendly honey, garlic, ginger and cabbage, so you can rest assured that it's working to your benefit.

MAKES 4 SERVINGS

⅓ cup (80 ml) coconut aminos

2 tbsp (30 ml) local honey

2 tbsp (30 ml) sesame oil

2 tbsp (18 g) minced garlic

1 tbsp (9 g) grated fresh ginger

2 tbsp (30 ml) extra-virgin olive oil

4 boneless, skinless organic chicken thighs or 2 organic boneless, skinless chicken breasts

Jicama Taco Shells (page 125)

Shredded green or red cabbage, as needed

In a small pot over medium heat, combine the coconut aminos, honey, sesame oil, garlic and ginger. Bring the mixture to a boil, then turn off the heat and set the pot aside.

Set the Instant Pot to Sauté at the hottest temperature. Once the Instant Pot says "Hot," add the olive oil and place the chicken in the pot, skin side down. Brown the chicken, about 3 minutes each side, then press the Cancel button.

Pour the sauce over the chicken and place the lid on the Instant Pot. Push the Manual button and cook for 10 minutes.

Place the chicken in the jicama shells and top the tacos with the cabbage. You may pick these up like a taco or cut them with a fork and knife.

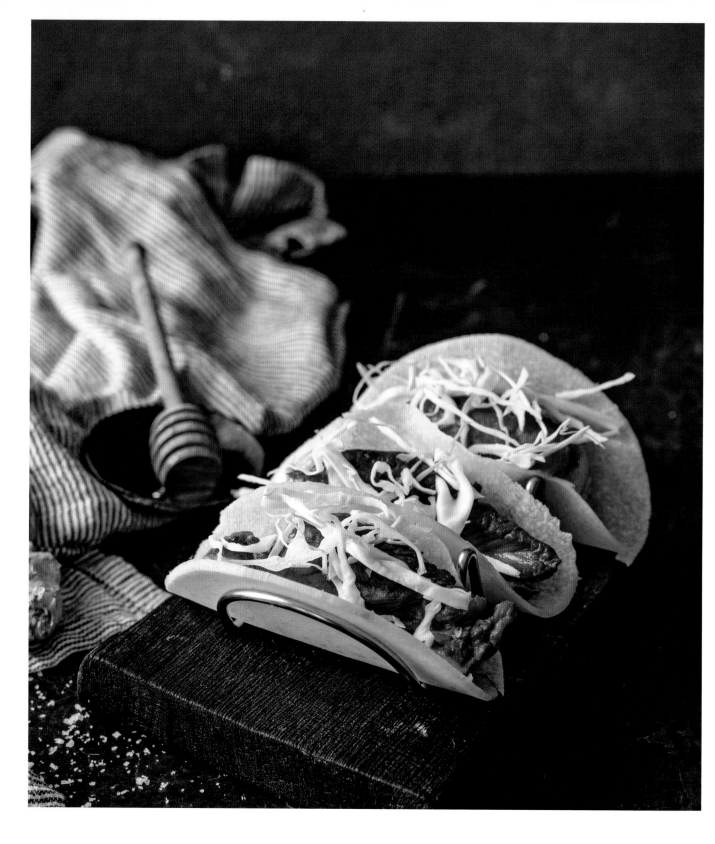

JICAMA TACO SHELLS

Jicama is a low-calorie, high-nutrient tuber that makes for a new twist in grain-free taco shells. Jicama is high in inulin, a soluble fiber, so it acts as a prebiotic, which is very supportive to the health of your gut. It's high in vitamin C, which is one of the most important nutrients for supporting those with histamine intolerance. It is also high in potassium, which is very supportive for the cardiovascular system.

MAKES APPROXIMATELY 12 TACO SHELLS

1 large firm, round jicama

Peel the jicama and slice it as thinly as possible. Soak the slices in cold water for 30 minutes.

Remove the jicama slices from the water and pat dry. Serve them right away with the Sesame-Ginger Chicken Tacos in Jicama Shells (page 123).

PORK CHOPS WITH FENNEL, ONION AND PEAR

Roasted pork is often paired with fennel in the Mediterranean. Here, the tender, juicy chops are accompanied by fresh thyme to help stabilize your mast cells and provide extra vitamin C and antioxidants. Pears are a delicious low-histamine fruit that complements this meal very well.

MAKES 4 SERVINGS

4 large organic pork chops

Sea salt, as needed

3 tbsp (45 ml) olive oil or melted coconut oil, divided

1 large Vidalia onion, thickly sliced

1 large head fennel, stems removed, thickly sliced

1 tbsp (2 g) plus 1 tsp fresh thyme leaves, divided

1 barely ripe pear (any variety), peeled and cut into moderately thick slices

Preheat the oven to 400°F (204°C).

Pound the pork chops lightly with a meat mallet and sprinkle the chops with the salt.

Heat 2 tablespoons (30 ml) of the oil in a large skillet over medium-high heat. Add the onion, fennel and ½ teaspoon of salt to the skillet and cook for 10 minutes. Sprinkle the mixture with 1 tablespoon (2 g) of the thyme and stir to combine, then remove the mixture from the skillet and transfer it to a large baking sheet.

Add the pork chops to the skillet and cook for 2 to 3 minutes on each side, or until they are browned. Remove the skillet from the heat and place the pork chops on top of the onion and fennel mixture. Spread the pear slices on top of the chops. Sprinkle the pork chops with the remaining 1 teaspoon of thyme.

Transfer the baking sheet to the oven and cook for 20 to 25 minutes, or until the pork is cooked through.

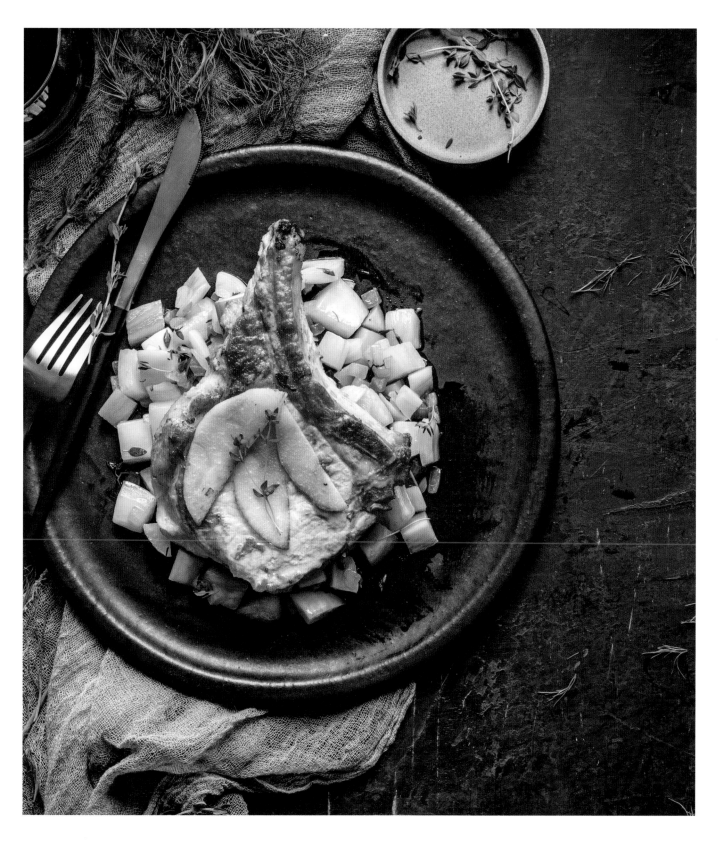

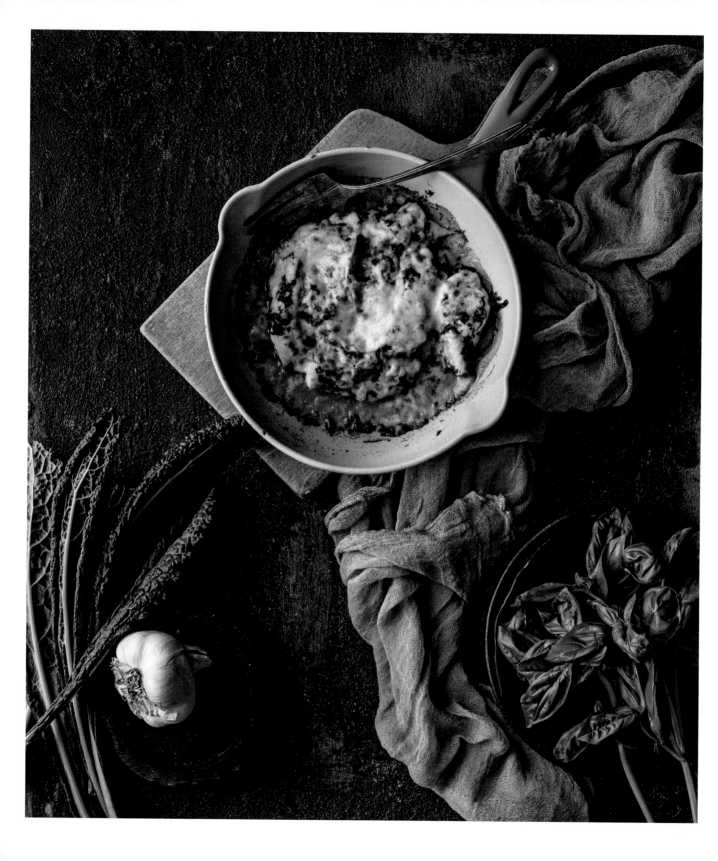

KALE PESTO CHEESY CHICKEN

This is a well-balanced dish that offers anti-inflammatory greens, lean protein and a satisfying portion of cheese to boot. I don't feel like I'm restricting my diet at all when I share this meal with my family. Mozzarella is a low-histamine cheese that is fine to indulge in from time to time. Raw mozzarella is even less inflammatory, so be sure to seek out that option in the area where you live.

MAKES 4 SERVINGS

½ cup (126 g) Kale Pesto (page 72)

2 boneless, skinless organic chicken breasts, thickly sliced

Shredded raw or grass-fed mozzarella cheese, as needed

Preheat the oven to 375°F (191°C). Coat the bottom of a medium roasting pan with a bit of the pesto.

Place the chicken in the roasting pan and cover it with the pesto. Cover the pan with foil and roast for 20 minutes.

Take the chicken out of the oven and cover it with the shredded mozzarella cheese. Place the pan back in the oven for 5 minutes.

Increase the oven temperature to broil and cook until the cheese is bubbling and lightly browned, 30 seconds to 1 minute.

PHASE 3: Omit the cheese and nuts from the pesto if you do not tolerate them.

CHICKEN, SWEET POTATO, APPLE AND BROCCOLI SKILLET

Here's a great recipe that's fast to put together and has a touch of sweetness, thanks to the apples and sweet potato, as well as plenty of flavor, thanks to the broth. This is fantastic to make during the week when your schedule might be more hectic. Almost all of the ingredients are antihistamine, including the broccoli, thanks to its natural quercetin content.

MAKES 4 SERVINGS

2 tbsp (30 ml) extra-virgin olive oil

1 lb (450 g) boneless, skinless organic chicken breast, cut into bite-size cubes

¾ tsp sea salt, divided

1 medium onion, coarsely chopped

2 cups (350 g) broccoli florets

1 medium sweet potato, peeled and cut into bite-size cubes

1 large or 2 small Gala apples, peeled, cored and cut into bite-size cubes

1 tbsp (2 g) coarsely chopped fresh thyme

3 cloves garlic, minced

¾ cup (180 ml) Low-Histamine Chicken Broth (page 71), divided

Heat the oil in a large skillet over medium-high heat. Add the chicken and sprinkle it with ¼ teaspoon of the sea salt. Cook until the chicken is lightly browned and cooked through, about 10 minutes, then remove it from the skillet and set aside.

Add the onion, broccoli and sweet potato to the skillet and sprinkle with the remaining ½ teaspoon of salt. Cook, stirring occasionally, until the onion is translucent and the sweet potato is soft, about 10 minutes.

Add the apple, thyme and garlic and cook for 1 minute. Add half the broth and cook for 3 minutes, or until the broth has evaporated. Transfer the chicken back to the skillet, add the remaining broth and cook for about 2 minutes.

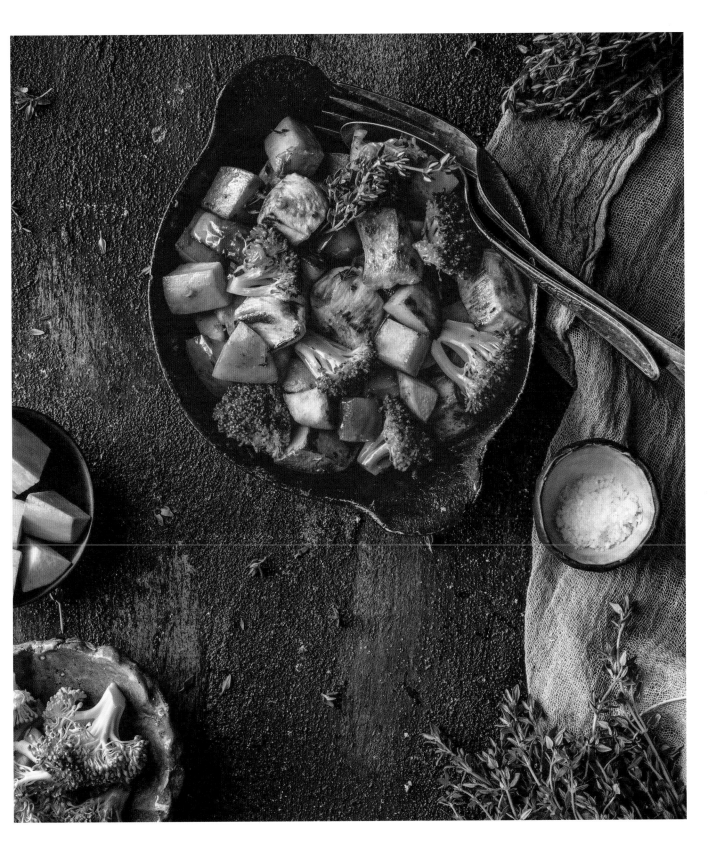

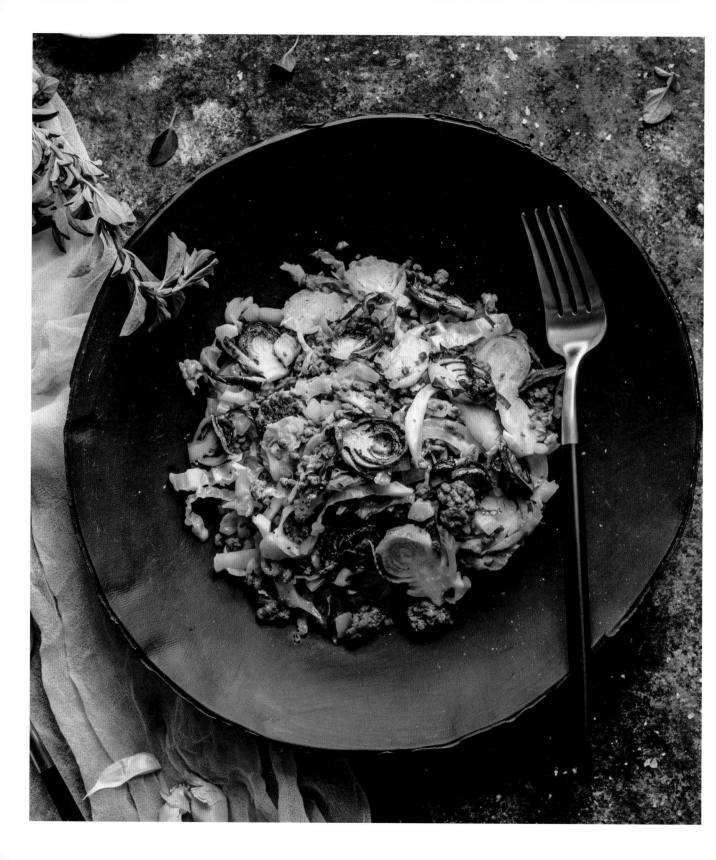

BEEF AND CABBAGE HASH

Here's another quick recipe that takes mere minutes to put together. The cabbage is soothing to the gut, so it's fantastic if you have leaky gut or you're working to maintain a healthy gut. The oregano, onion and garlic add a therapeutic antihistamine kick.

MAKES 4 SERVINGS

1 lb (450 g) grass-fed beef or ground organic turkey

½ tbsp (1 g) finely chopped fresh oregano

¼ tsp sea salt, plus more as needed

2 tbsp (28 g) grass-fed butter

½ large head green or red cabbage, thinly sliced

1 large onion, coarsely chopped

½ lb (225 g) Brussels sprouts, shredded

4 cloves garlic, minced

In a medium skillet over medium-high heat, combine the beef, oregano and ¼ teaspoon of salt. Cook until the beef is cooked through, about 10 minutes, and then remove it from the skillet and set aside.

Wipe out the skillet and return it to medium-high heat. Add the butter to the skillet and let it melt. Add the cabbage, onion, Brussels sprouts and additional salt and cook for 5 minutes, stirring frequently. Add the garlic and cook for 5 more minutes, until the cabbage and Brussels sprouts are wilted.

Transfer the beef back to the skillet and stir to combine. Cook for 1 to 2 minutes and serve.

POACHED CHICKEN AND GREEN BEANS IN GINGER BROTH

A simple recipe that's perfect for colder months, this delicious chicken plate is Paleo, keto, Whole30 and AIP-friendly. Here's another instance when the broth you made earlier saves time preparing antihistamine herbs and spices. The ginger adds an Asian touch.

MAKES 4 SERVINGS

2 tbsp (18 g) peeled, grated fresh ginger

4 scallions, finely chopped

2 tbsp (30 ml) coconut aminos

4 cups (960 ml) Low-Histamine Chicken Broth (page 71)

4 boneless, skinless organic chicken breasts

10 oz (280 g) fresh green beans, trimmed

Combine the ginger, scallions, coconut aminos and broth in a large wok or deep skillet over medium-high heat. Simmer the mixture for 3 minutes.

Add the chicken and cook it for 6 minutes on each side, then remove it from the wok and set aside.

Add the green beans and cook until they are tender, about 5 minutes.

Divide the broth and green beans among four shallow bowls, place the chicken on top and serve.

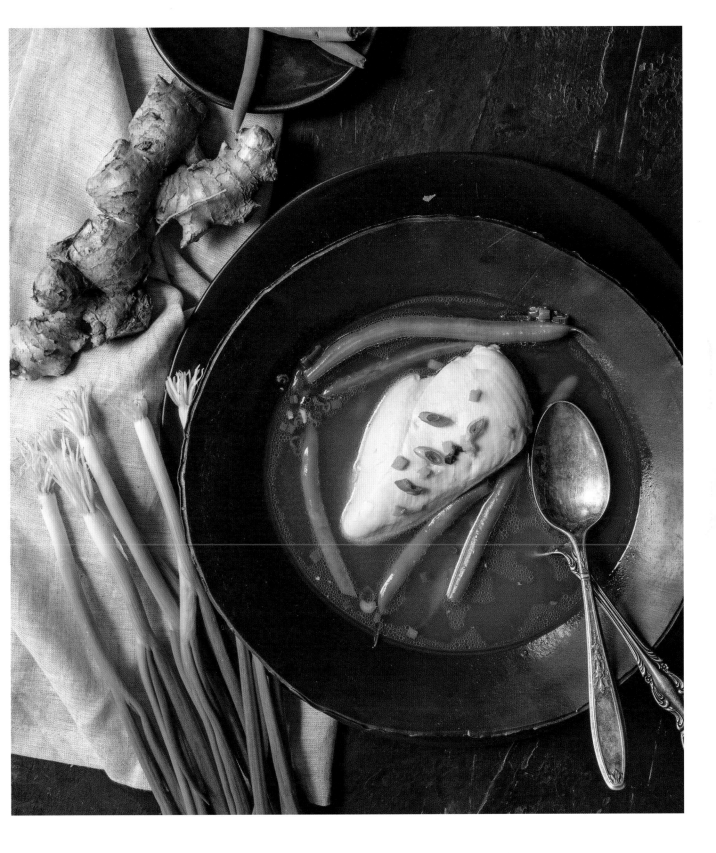

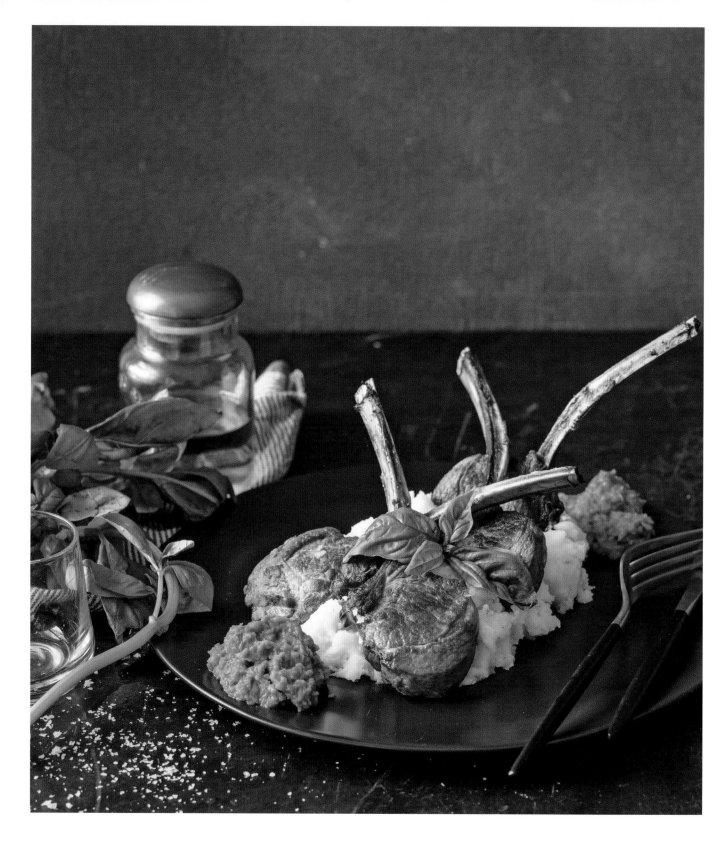

LAMB LOLLIPOPS WITH BASIL AND PEA PUREE

I've adapted this recipe to include basil for extra antihistamine power. I really love how it turned out: creamy, filling and wholesome. Most people can tolerate coconut and the rest of the ingredients in this recipe, making it a great neutral main dish for any type of evening.

MAKES 4 SERVINGS

PEA PUREE

3 large white potatoes, peeled

4 tbsp (56 g) grass-fed butter

¾ cup (180 ml) coconut cream

Sea salt, to taste

2 cups (300 g) peas, thawed if frozen

3 tbsp (6 g) coarsely chopped fresh basil

LAMB

2 tbsp (30 ml) extra-virgin olive oil, plus more as needed

4 organic lamb lollipops

2 tbsp (4 g) coarsely chopped fresh basil

Sea salt, to taste

To make the pea puree, place the potatoes in a large pot, cover them with cold water and bring the water to a boil over medium-high heat. Cook the potatoes for about 15 minutes, until they are soft. Remove the pot from the heat, drain the water from the potatoes and let them cool slightly.

Transfer the potatoes back to the pot and mash them well with a potato masher. Add the butter, coconut cream and salt and blend with a hand mixer or whisk until smooth.

Place the peas in a small pot, cover them with cold water and bring the water to a boil over medium-high heat. Cook the peas for 5 minutes, then drain them and allow them to cool slightly.

Place the peas, basil and 4 tablespoons (53 g) of the mashed potatoes in a food processor and process until smooth. Add the pea mixture to the remaining potato mixture in the pot and stir to combine. Cook over low heat until the puree is warm.

To make the lamb, heat the oil in a medium skillet over medium-high heat. Coat each side of the lamb with additional oil and sprinkle each side with the basil and salt. Place the lamb in the skillet and cook for about 5 minutes on each side.

Serve the lamb over the pea puree.

Sides can spice up any main dish and provide variation. You might also like to serve yourself or your family a meal that purely consists of side dishes one day. They are also perfect for parties and potlucks. Just make sure you eat before you go out to events that might have foods you're trying to avoid! Unless, that is, you're going to a special antihistamine event.

ROSEMARY AND SALT BREAD

Contrary to popular belief, it is absolutely possible to enjoy bread without any gluten. This homemade loaf is slightly sweet and salty and makes the perfect canvas for pesto, hummus or a little butter—it also shines as an accompaniment to any of the soup recipes in this book.

MAKES 12 SERVINGS

1 cup (96 g) almond flour (page 67)

¼ cup (31 g) tapioca flour (page 66)

¼ cup (31 g) cassava flour (page 66)

1 tsp aluminum-free baking powder

½ tsp sea salt

3 large pasture-raised eggs

⅓ cup (82 g) unsweetened applesauce

1 tbsp (2 g) finely chopped fresh rosemary

Preheat the oven to 350°F (177°C). Line a standard-size bread pan with parchment paper.

In a large bowl, combine the almond flour, tapioca flour, cassava flour, baking powder and salt.

In a medium bowl, combine the eggs and applesauce.

Add the egg mixture to the flour mixture and combine with a spoon or whisk. Fold in the rosemary and pour the batter into the prepared bread pan. Bake for 55 minutes, or until a toothpick inserted into the center of the bread comes out clean.

PHASE 3: Use 1 cup (122 g) of cassava flour and ½ cup (62 g) of tapioca flour. Use ½ cup (123 g) of unsweetened applesauce and omit the eggs (or you can try 3 large pasture-raised yolks without the whites).

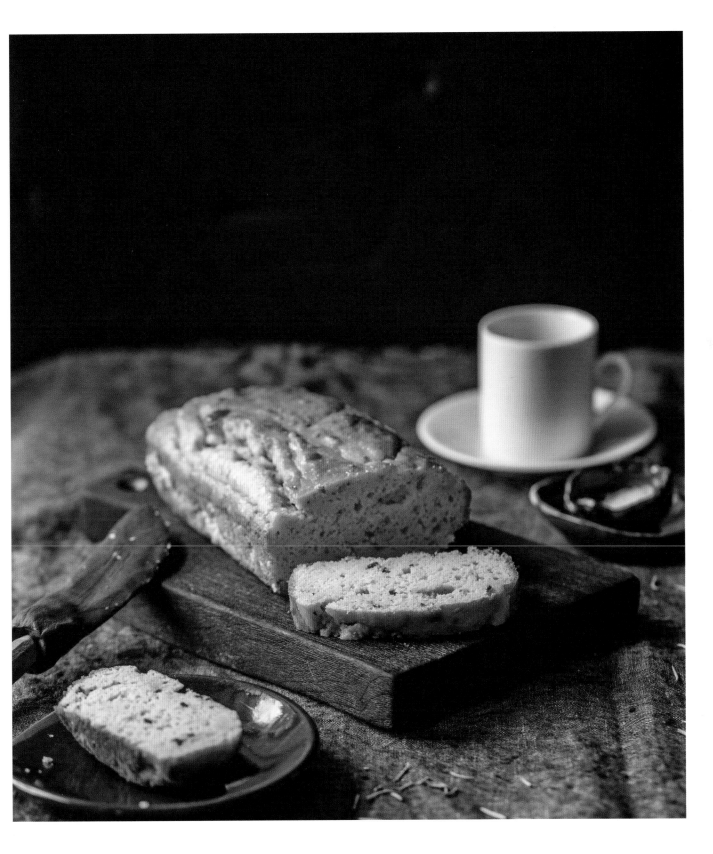

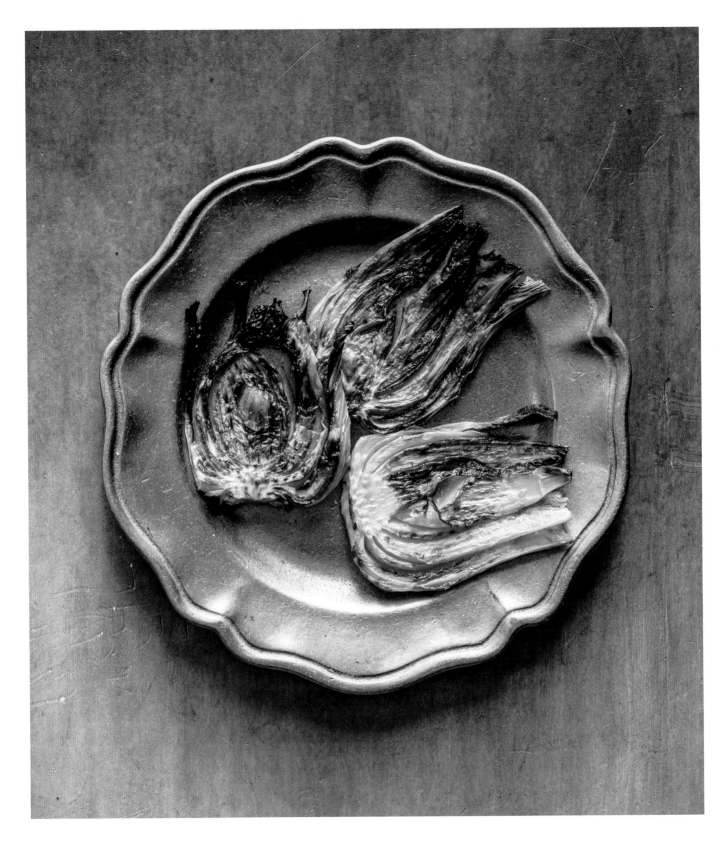

CARAMELIZED FENNEL

Fennel is an antihistamine food with a very distinct, fresh, licorice-like flavor that really doesn't need an accompaniment. It is also high in fiber, potassium, folate, vitamin C and other important nutrients. When cooked just enough, fennel is soft and very satisfying.

MAKES 4 SERVINGS

2 large heads fennel

Extra-virgin olive oil, as needed

Sea salt, as needed

Preheat the oven to 400°F (204°C). Line a large baking sheet with parchment paper.

Trim the green fronds from the fennel and discard them. Remove the ends of the fennel heads and place the fennel end-side down on a worksurface. Slice them into ¼-inch (6-mm)-thick pieces. Place the fennel pieces on the prepared baking sheet.

Drizzle the fennel with the desired amount of oil (I recommend about 2 tablespoons [30 ml]) and toss to coat. Sprinkle the fennel with the salt and bake for 30 to 40 minutes, until the ends are browned.

MASHED JAPANESE SWEET POTATOES

All naturally purple foods contain more antioxidants than their less brightly colored counterparts. Sweet potatoes are no different. The Japanese sweet potato is one of the most potent antihistamine foods. It also makes this dish really stand out at the dinner table.

MAKES 4 SERVINGS

4 medium Japanese sweet potatoes, peeled and cubed

2 tbsp (28 g) grass-fed butter

⅛ tsp sea salt

Unsweetened vanilla almond or coconut milk (for a sweet dish) or broth (page 71; for a savory dish), as needed

Place the sweet potatoes in a large pot. Cover them with cold water and bring the water to a boil over medium-high heat. Cook until the potatoes are tender, about 15 minutes. Drain the water and add the butter, salt and milk or broth. Blend with a hand mixer until the potatoes are smooth.

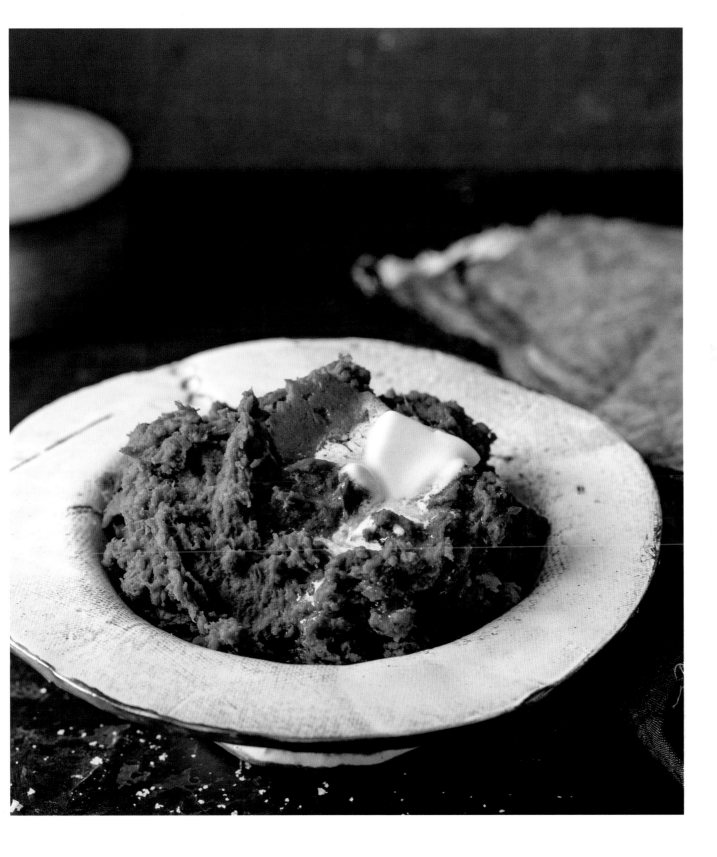

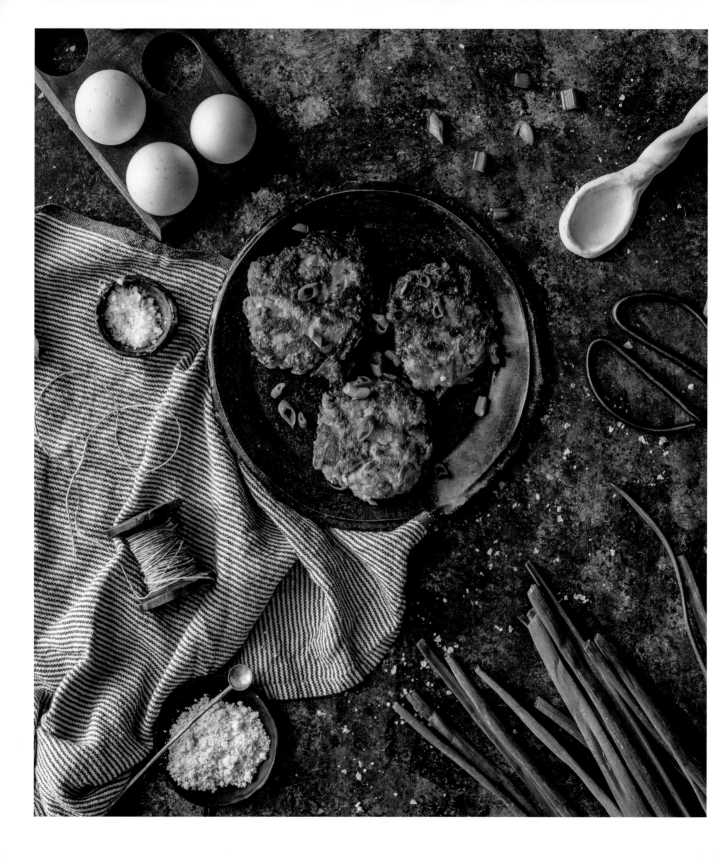

SWEET POTATO LATKES

These sweet potato pancakes are a variation of the traditional potato pancakes the Ashkenazi Jews have prepared as part of the Hanukkah festival since the mid-1880s. These fritters are a delight for the senses and have added garlic to make sure they are antihistamine.

MAKES 4 SERVINGS

2 medium sweet potatoes, peeled and grated

4 cloves garlic, minced

3 large pasture-raised eggs, beaten

2 tbsp (12 g) almond flour (page 67)

1 tsp sea salt

Extra-virgin olive oil, as needed

Coarsely chopped scallions, as needed

In a large bowl, combine the sweet potatoes, garlic, eggs, flour and salt until evenly mixed. Form the mixture into thin patties.

Heat a generous amount of oil in a medium skillet over medium-high heat. Fry the patties for about 3 minutes on each side, or until they are golden brown. Sprinkle the latkes with the scallions and serve.

PHASE 3: Replace almond flour with tapioca flour if you do not tolerate nuts.

CRISPY CARROTS AND GARLIC

Most root vegetables are low-histamine foods, but the vitamin A that carrots provide make them a little more special than the rest. This side would be nice to serve alongside any main plate in this book.

MAKES 2 SERVINGS

4 large carrots, peeled lengthwise into ribbons

3 tbsp (45 ml) extra-virgin olive oil

4 cloves garlic, minced

¼ tsp sea salt

Preheat the oven to 325°F (163°C).

In a medium bowl, combine the carrots, oil, garlic and salt and toss to coat. Spread the carrots on a medium baking sheet in an even layer. Bake for 30 minutes, or until the carrots' edges are crispy.

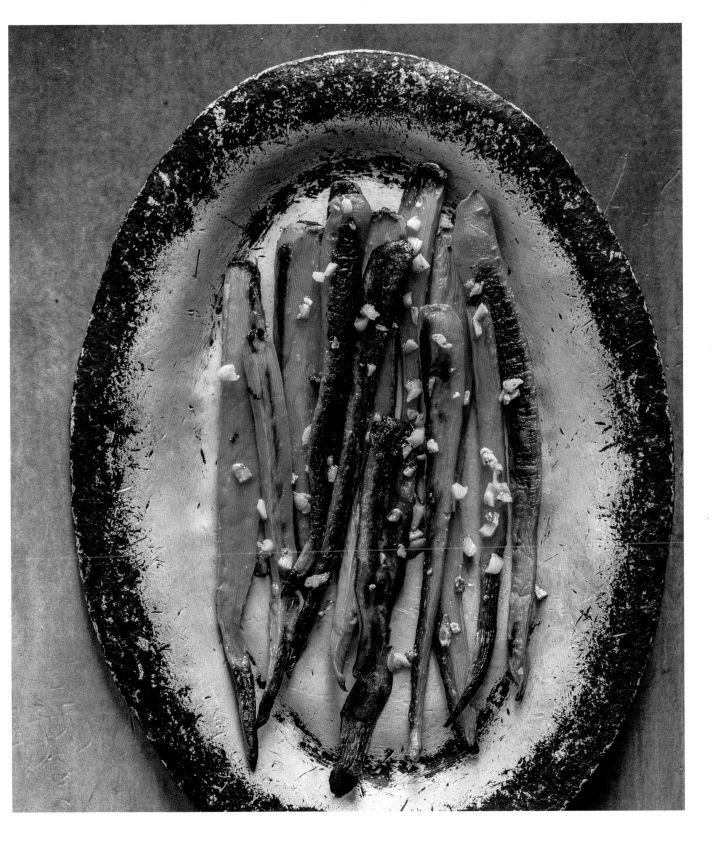

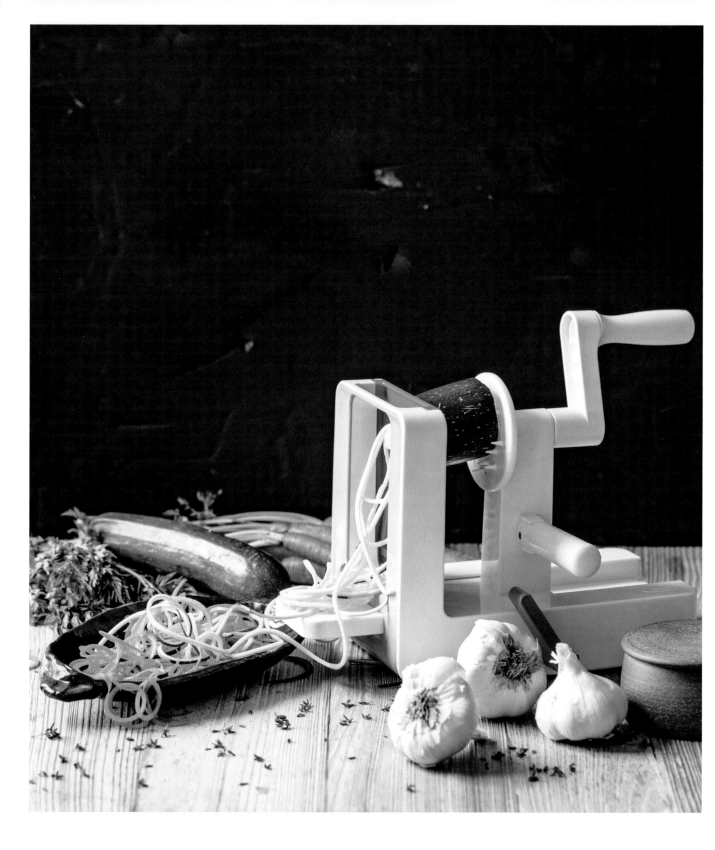

ZUCCHINI AND CARROT "NOODLES"

Flavor and texture are everything when you're on a restricted diet. This recipe should do a good job at tricking your brain into thinking you're eating grain-based noodles! Try it and let me know what you think.

MAKES 4 SERVINGS

1 tbsp (15 ml) extra-virgin olive oil

4 large carrots, peeled lengthwise into ribbons

4 large zucchini, peeled lengthwise into ribbons

5 cloves garlic, minced

1 tbsp (14 g) grass-fed butter

Coarsely chopped fresh thyme

Heat the oil in a large skillet over medium heat. Add the carrots and zucchini and cook for 5 minutes, adding the garlic during the final minute and mixing well. Add the butter and thyme and mix well.

GARLIC AND CHIVE BUTTER BRUSSELS SPROUTS

Eating a lot of vegetables can be a challenge for many, but not when they are topped with a lavish dollop of herb butter! This is another dish that is perfect for sharing.

MAKES 4 SERVINGS

BRUSSELS SPROUTS

1 lb (450 g) Brussels sprouts, ends trimmed, halved

2 tbsp (30 ml) extra-virgin olive oil

Sea salt, to taste

BUTTER SAUCE

4 tbsp (56 g) grass-fed butter

1½ tbsp (14 g) minced garlic

1½ tbsp (3 g) finely chopped fresh chives

Preheat the oven to 400°F (204°C).

To make the Brussels sprouts, place the Brussels sprouts on a medium baking sheet and coat them with the oil and salt, tossing with your hands to combine. Cook the Brussels sprouts for 30 minutes, or until lightly browned.

To make the butter sauce, melt the butter in a small pot over medium-low heat. Add the garlic and chives and cook for about 3 minutes, stirring frequently.

Remove the Brussels sprouts from the oven and spoon the butter sauce on top.

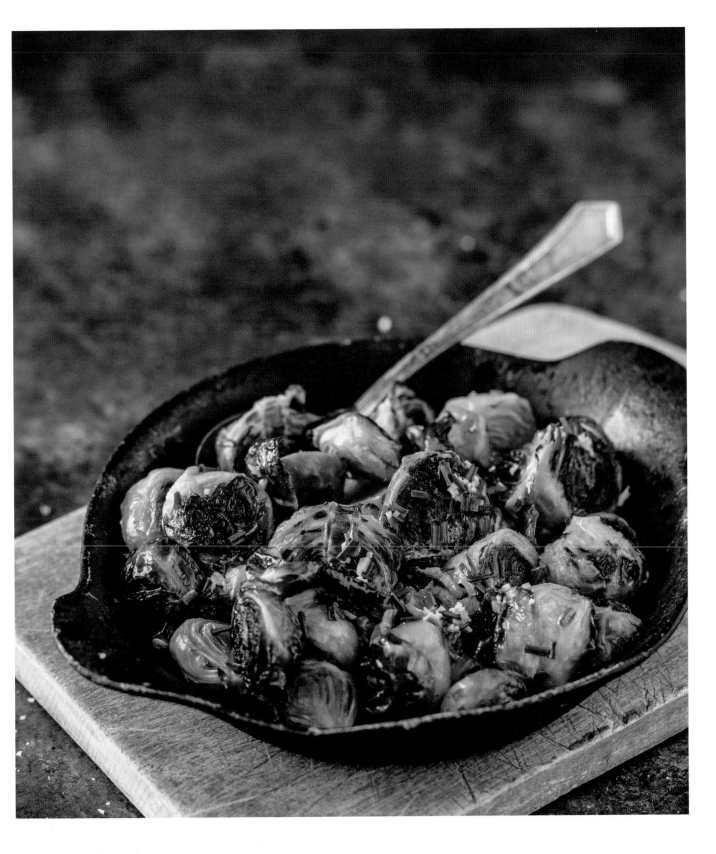

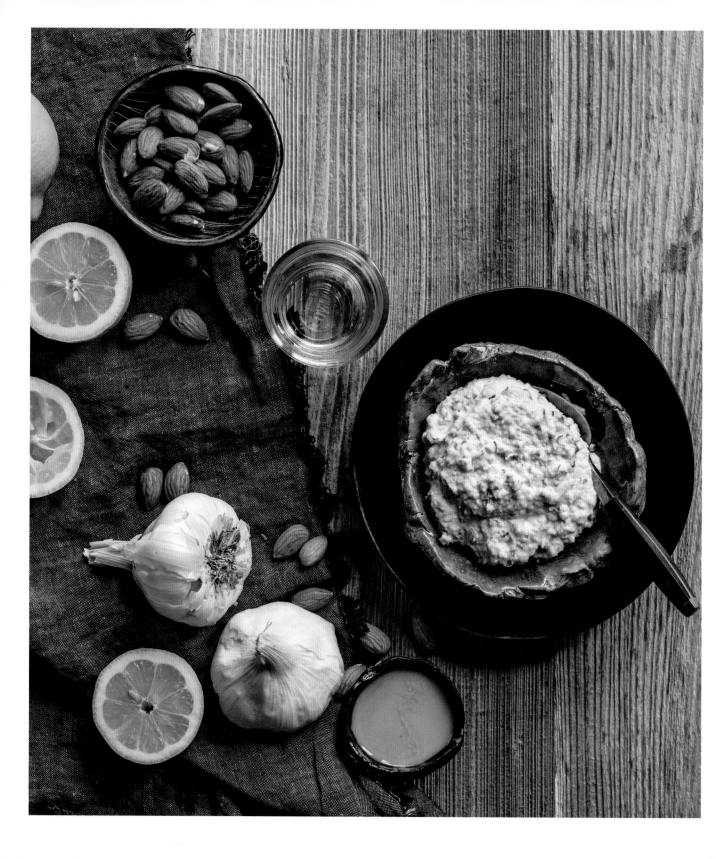

ALMOND HUMMUS

You never know what might be included in the ingredients of a container of store-bought hummus, but this hummus is guaranteed to be clean, nourishing and tasty. It can be used as a dip for veggies or spread on low-histamine bread.

MAKES 8 TO 10 SERVINGS

2 cups (340 g) raw almonds, soaked in water for at least 4 hours

½ cup (112 g) tahini

3 to 4 cloves garlic, coarsely chopped

2 tsp (6 g) ground cumin

1 tsp sea salt

⅓ cup (80 ml) warm water

½ cup (120 ml) extra-virgin olive oil

Juice of 3 lemons (optional)

Place the almonds, tahini, garlic, cumin, salt, water, oil and lemon juice, if using, in a food processor and process on high speed until the ingredients are smooth. Add more oil or water until the desired consistency is reached.

PHASE 3: Omit the almonds and use 1 head of cauliflower, cut into florets, steamed and cooled.

DRINKS AND DESSERTS

Welcome to my favorite section of the book: the drinks and desserts. When you're on a low-histamine diet, I want you to stay hydrated in creative ways and to make sure you're consuming desserts once in a while as a treat. This will make it so much easier to stay on target without feeling like you're being deprived. Here are my favorite recipes for you to try.

CREAMY MANGO SMOOTHIE

Never tried adding cauliflower to a smoothie? I was skeptical at first, too, until I tried it. This is a satisfyingly sneaky way of adding more vegetables to your day while also making your smoothie creamier. You won't taste any cruciferous vegetables, I promise. This is a fragrant, milky, creamy, antihistamine smoothie others will want to try.

MAKES 1 SERVING

½ cup (123 g) frozen cubed mango

½ cup (90 g) frozen cauliflower florets

¼ cup (41 g) chia seeds

1 tsp preservative-free vanilla extract

1 cup (240 ml) dairy-free milk

Ice cubes, if needed

Combine the mango, cauliflower, chia seeds, vanilla, milk and ice cubes in a blender and blend until smooth.

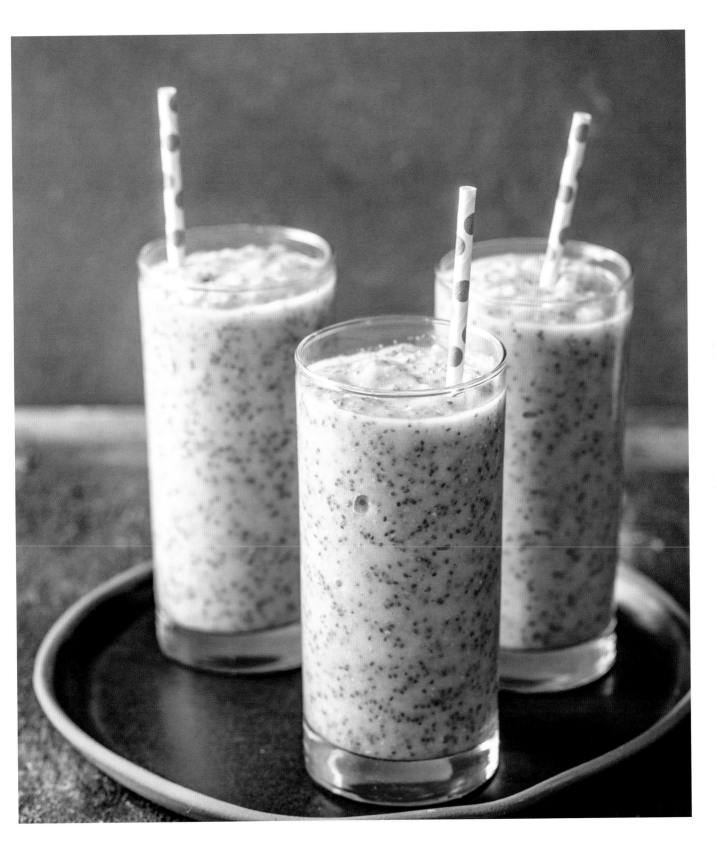

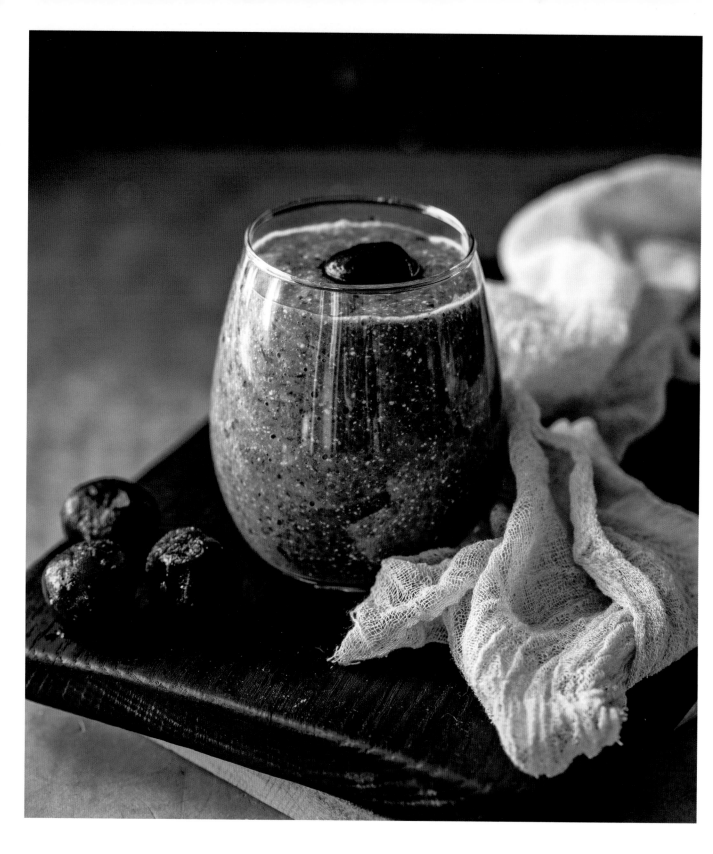

OVERNIGHT CHERRY–CHIA SMOOTHIE

I like to make my cooking time as productive as possible and sometimes make breakfast for the next day while I'm making dinner. Some breakfast recipes can also be served as dessert, though others, like this one, have the best flavor and texture when allowed to sit in the refrigerator for at least 4 hours. Cherries are high in quercetin, which reduces histamine levels in the body. Chia seeds are beautifully soothing for the gut and rich in antioxidants, fiber, iron and calcium.

MAKES 1 SERVING

1 serving Chia Seed Pudding (page 79), prior to being chilled

½ cup (80 g) fresh or frozen cherries

Combine the pudding and cherries in a blender and blend until smooth. Pour the smoothie into a Mason jar. Chill the smoothie overnight or for at least 4 hours.

APPLE, CARROT AND GINGER JUICE

Vegetables that are high in vitamin A can help control allergic reactions, and consuming them raw and as juices allows you to receive all the benefits they have to offer. This juice contains a large dose of vitamin A–rich carrots, as well as antihistamine compounds thanks to the apples and ginger.

MAKES 1 SERVING

6 carrots

1 large green apple

1 (1-inch [2.5-cm]) piece fresh ginger, peeled

Process the carrots, apple and ginger in a juicer and serve immediately.

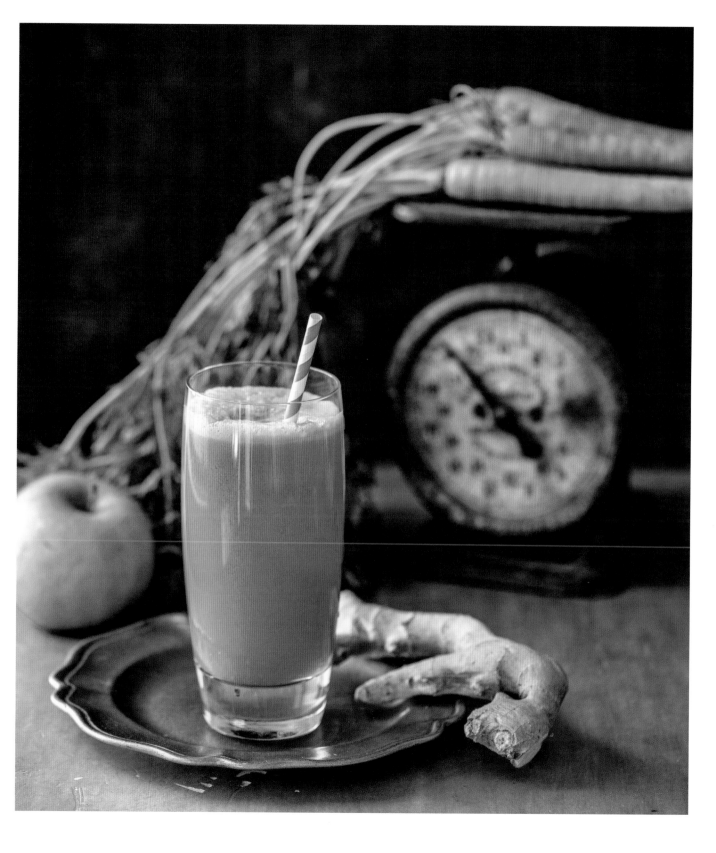

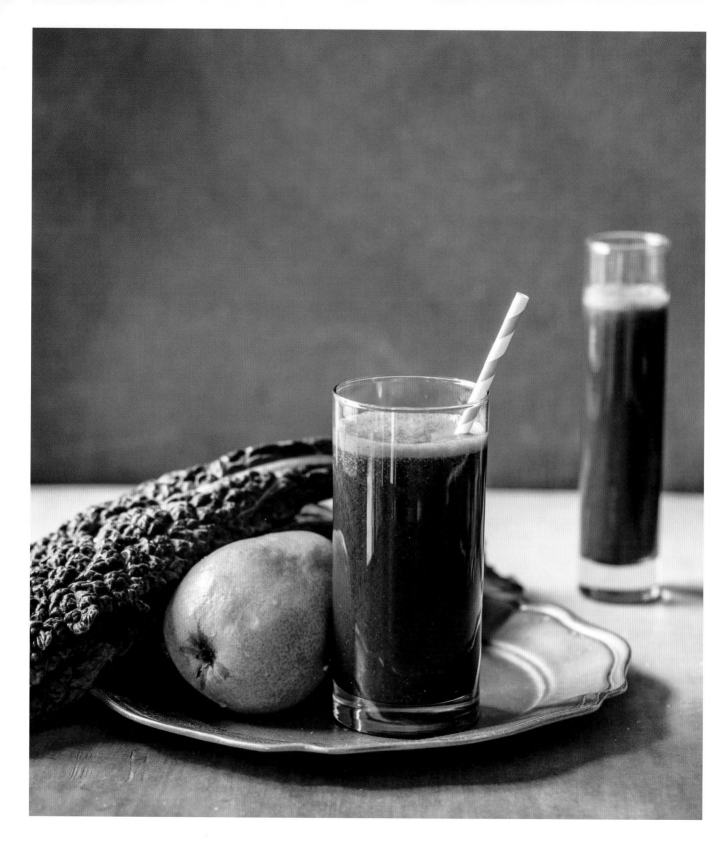

KALE, PEAR, CUCUMBER AND CELERY JUICE

I'm always amazed at how many vegetables I can add to a juice that contains fruit without it affecting the taste. Sweet pears are neutral, the cucumber is refreshing and light, the kale is antihistamine and the celery is too! Celery contains quercetin and luteolin, as well as being anti-inflammatory and healing to the digestive tract.

MAKES 1 SERVING

1 medium bunch kale, with stems

2 large ribs celery

½ medium cucumber

1½ pears

Process the kale, celery, cucumber and pears in a juicer and serve immediately.

ROSEMARY SHORTBREAD

With this shortbread, you'll be feeding the good bacteria in your gut with the cassava flour while keeping histamine low thanks to the rosemary. This bread also smells wonderful as it's baking.

MAKES 6 SERVINGS

⅓ cup (48 g) maple sugar

1 tsp preservative-free vanilla

¾ cup (92 g) cassava flour (page 66)

1 tsp coarsely chopped fresh rosemary

½ cup (115 g) cold salted grass-fed butter, cut into chunks

Preheat the oven to 325°F (163°C). Grease a 9-inch (23-cm) round pie pan.

Place the sugar, vanilla, flour, rosemary and butter in a food processor and pulse for about 10 seconds, or just until everything is combined. Remove the dough from the processor and form it into a ball, making sure everything is sticking together well and that it is not flaky.

Place the dough into the prepared pie pan and press it into a thin layer. Bake for 30 minutes, or until the shortbread is golden on the edges.

Let the shortbread cool for 5 minutes before cutting.

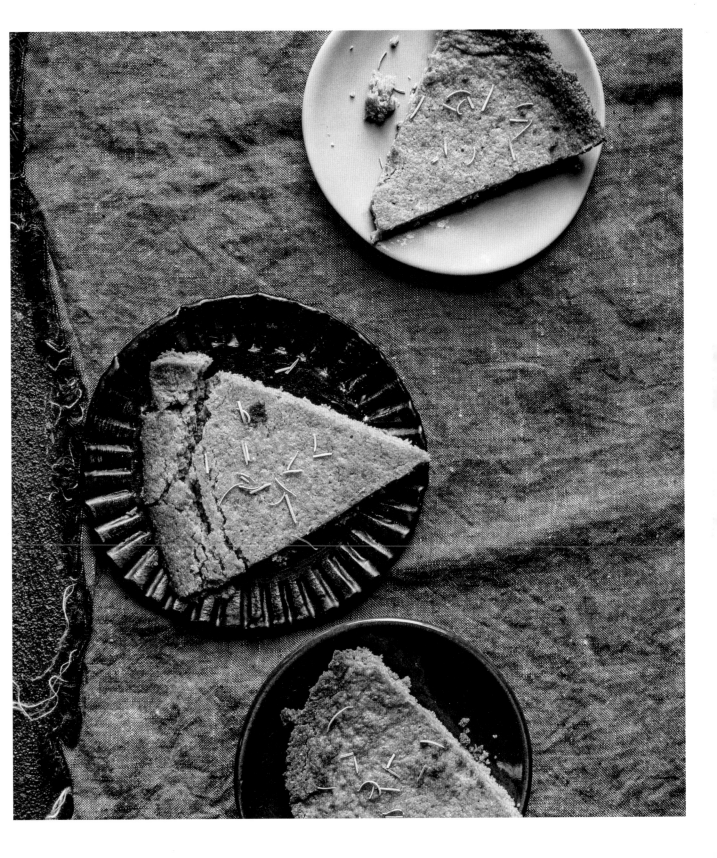

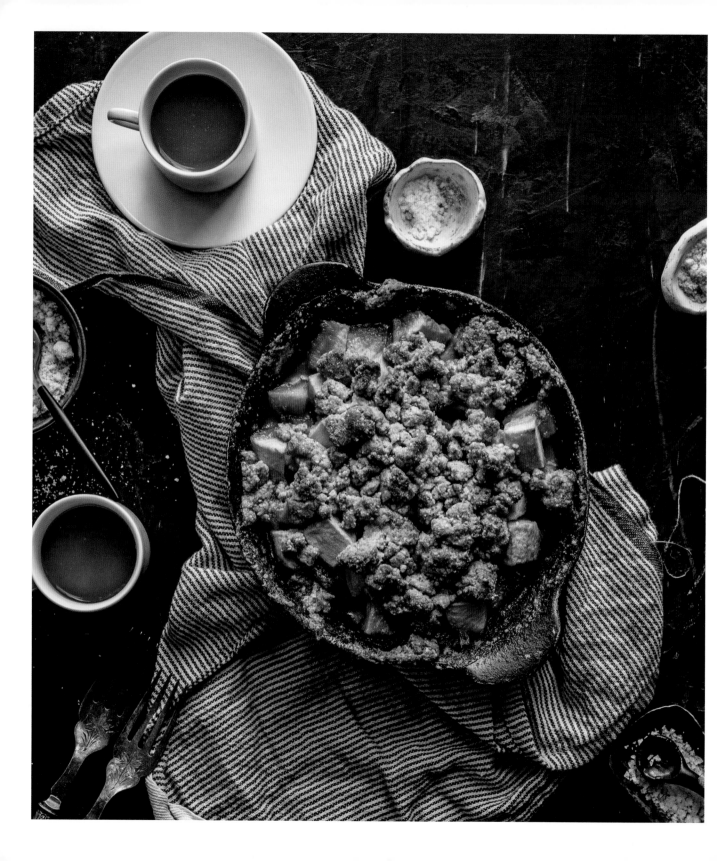

APPLE CRISP

Apples taste fantastic raw and crispy, but cooked apples take on a whole different quality. They're recommended for histamine intolerance thanks to their natural quercetin content, and here they're dressed up with a crumb topping.

MAKES 8 SERVINGS

FILLING

¼ cup (60 ml) full-fat coconut milk

2 tsp (10 ml) preservative-free vanilla extract

2 tbsp (30 ml) maple syrup

1 tbsp (9 g) maple sugar

½ tsp tapioca or arrowroot powder

4 cups (440 g) peeled and sliced Gala apples

CRUMB TOPPING

4 tbsp (56 g) room-temperature grass-fed butter or coconut oil

¼ cup (28 g) coconut flour (page 67)

½ cup (48 g) almond flour (page 67)

2 tbsp (18 g) maple sugar

⅛ tsp sea salt

4 tbsp (32 g) finely chopped pecans or almonds (optional)

Preheat the oven to 375°F (191°C). Grease a 9-inch (23-cm) pie pan or an 8 x 8-inch (20 x 20–cm) baking dish with coconut oil.

To make the filling, combine the coconut milk, vanilla, maple syrup, maple sugar and tapioca powder in a medium bowl. Add the apples and coat them with the milk mixture.

To make the crumb topping, combine the butter, coconut flour, almond flour, maple sugar, salt and pecans, if using, in a small bowl. Mix with a fork or your hands until the mixture is crumbly.

Pour the apple mixture into the prepared pie pan and bake for 30 minutes. Remove the pie pan from the oven and sprinkle the crumb topping over the apples. Bake for about 20 minutes, or until the apples are soft and the topping is browned. Serve warm.

VANILLA-SOAKED PEARS

This is a recipe that's quick to put together when you have all the ingredients on hand. I often make it last-minute for this reason when craving something sweet and antihistamine, criteria that, thanks to the pears, this recipe meets.

MAKES 4 SERVINGS

1 cup (240 ml) water

¼ cup (36 g) maple or coconut sugar

½ vanilla bean, split and scraped

2 semi-ripe Bartlett pears, halved and seeded

Place the water, maple sugar and vanilla bean in a medium pot over low heat and cook, stirring frequently, until the sugar is dissolved, 3 to 4 minutes. Add the pears and simmer until they are soft, about 5 minutes.

Divide the pears among four bowls and pour the sauce over the top.

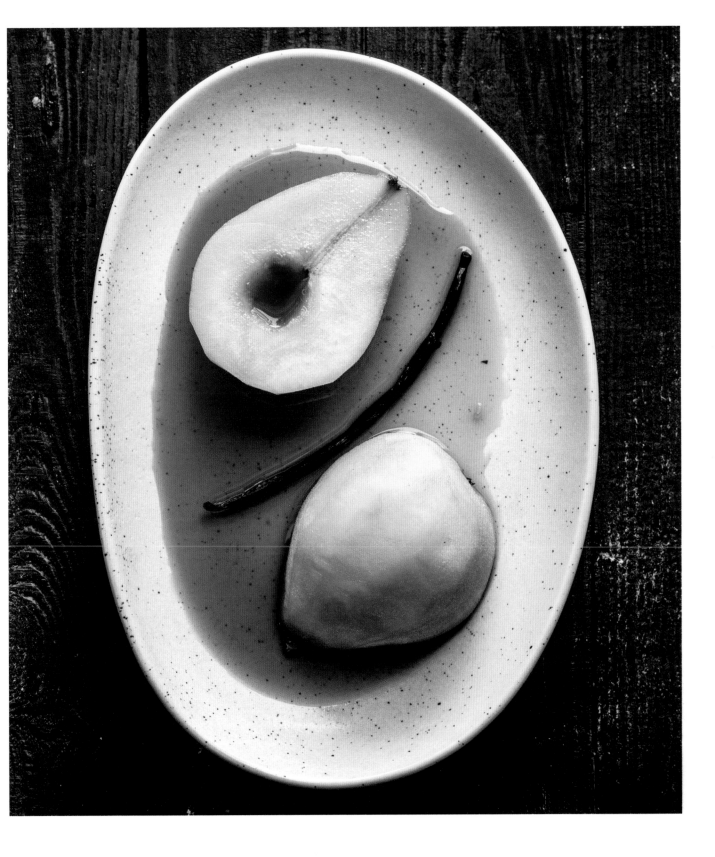

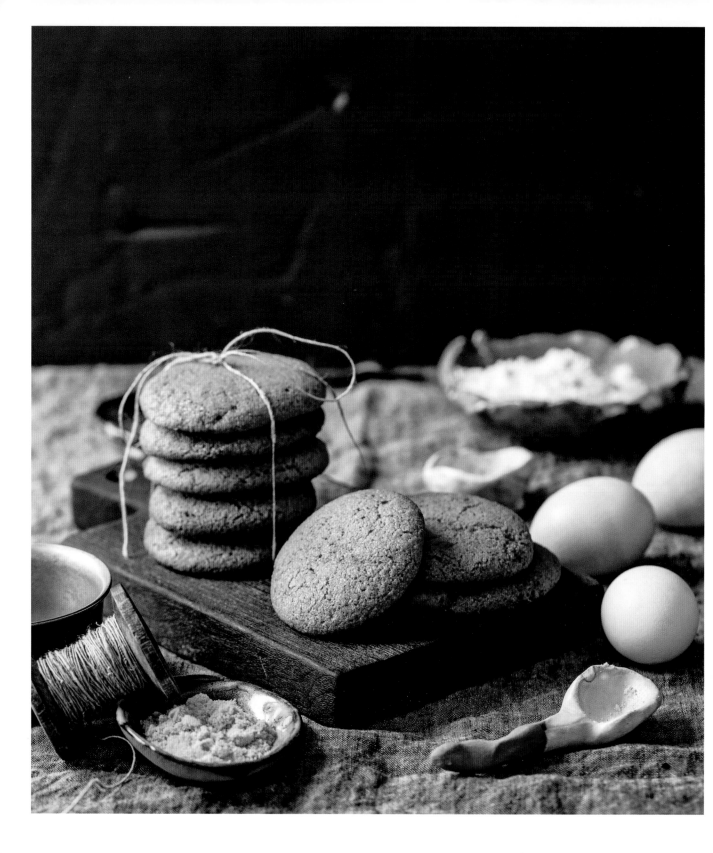

ANTIHISTAMINE GINGER COOKIES

Ginger is anti-inflammatory and stabilizes mast cells. So why not make cookies? This easy, popular recipe will allow you to share food with anyone who might come to visit. These cookies are high in good fat, so you won't have to worry about eating one too many.

MAKES 15 COOKIES

1 cup (96 g) almond flour (page 67)

½ cup (63 g) tapioca flour (page 66)

¼ cup (28 g) coconut flour (page 67)

½ cup (72 g) maple sugar

1 tsp baking soda

1½ tsp (5 g) ground ginger

½ tsp sea salt

1 large pasture-raised egg or 2 large pasture-raised egg yolks if you do not tolerate egg whites

3 tbsp (45 ml) blackstrap molasses

½ cup (115 g) coconut oil, melted

Preheat the oven to 350°F (177°C). Line a large baking sheet with parchment paper.

In a large bowl, combine the almond flour, tapioca flour, coconut flour, maple sugar, baking soda, ginger and salt.

In a small bowl, combine the egg, molasses and coconut oil. Add the egg mixture to the flour mixture and combine with a hand mixer or spoon.

Scoop out a heaping tablespoon (15 g) of dough, roll it into a ball and place it on the prepared baking sheet; repeat this process with the remaining dough. You should get 15 cookies.

Bake the cookies for 15 minutes, or until browned at the edges. If needed, push the cookies down slightly with a spoon to help flatten them about halfway through the baking time.

PHASE 3: Substitute the almond flour for 1 cup (122 g) of cassava flour or tigernut flour.

DRESSINGS

When it comes to salad dressings, those of us who are intolerant to high-histamine foods can really struggle because most vinegars are high in histamine. White distilled vinegar happens to be the lowest-histamine vinegar and apple cider vinegar is a close second. Some can tolerate these, while others can't. You will want to experiment with these and see which one you tolerate best, even trying lemon in their place if you tolerate that. I find that salad dressing tends to be okay when made ahead of time and stored in the refrigerator for up to three days. Some of you may need to make dressing fresh with each salad if you are still reacting strongly to most foods. If so, just reduce the oil to about ¼ cup (60 ml) and the vinegar to about 1 tablespoon (15 ml) and add small amounts of the other ingredients.

TARRAGON VINAIGRETTE

Tarragon goes well with pork, chicken and fish. It also stabilizes mast cells and is one of the richest antioxidant herbs, helping calm inflammation in the digestive tract.

MAKES 1¼ CUPS (300 ML)

¼ cup (60 ml) organic white distilled vinegar

1 cup (240 ml) extra-light olive oil

1 packed cup (42 g) fresh tarragon

1 tsp sea salt

In a blender, combine the vinegar, oil, tarragon and salt. Blend until there are no pieces of tarragon remaining. Keep the dressing refrigerated for up to 36 hours (you may be able to go up to 72 hours).

APPLE CIDER VINAIGRETTE

If you can tolerate apple cider vinegar, you're going to love this vinaigrette, which has all the sweet, salty and acidic flavors to make a fantastic, balanced dressing for any antihistamine salad. If you cannot tolerate apple cider vinegar, try using white distilled vinegar in its place.

MAKES 1¼ TO 1½ CUPS (300 TO 360 ML)

¼ to ½ cup (60 to 120 ml) apple cider vinegar

1 cup (240 ml) extra-virgin olive oil

1 tsp local honey

1 tsp sea salt

Combine the vinegar, oil, honey and salt in a large Mason jar and shake vigorously until the ingredients are incorporated. Keep the dressing refrigerated for up to 36 hours (you may be able to go up to 72 hours).

GINGER DRESSING

This warming, antihistamine ginger dressing can be drizzled over some fresh watercress or arugula or over any basic vegetable dish, especially on a cold night when you're not feeling particularly energetic. Be sure to blend it well or grate the ginger finely to ensure the texture of your dressing isn't fibrous.

MAKES 1¼ CUPS (300 ML)

1 cup (240 ml) extra-virgin olive oil

¼ cup (60 ml) distilled white vinegar

1 tsp grated ginger

1 tsp local honey

Combine the oil, vinegar, ginger and honey in a large Mason jar or blender and shake or blend thoroughly. Keep refrigerated for up to 36 hours (you may be able to go up to 72 hours).

Antihistamine Meal Plan

	DAY 1	DAY 2	DAY 3	DAY 4	DAY 5	DAY 6
BREAKFAST	"PB and J" Chia Pudding	Spiced-Up Eggs Over Greens	Creamy Mango Smoothie	Kale and Sweet Potato Egg Muffins	Apple Bread	Asparagus and Red Potato Frittata
LUNCH	Chicken Sausage, Kale and Sweet Potato Soup with optional slice of Rosemary and Salt Bread	Apple, Pecan and Chicken Arugula Salad	Rosemary and Garlic Lamb Burger with Caramelized Fennel	Kale and Onion Chicken Patty Wrap with Mashed Japanese Sweet Potatoes	Artichoke Soup with optional slice of Rosemary and Salt Bread	Chicken and Mango Salad
DINNER	Pork Medallions with Shaved Brussels and Carrots	Instant Pot Chicken with Gravy and Cauliflower Mash	Antihistamine Chicken Stir-Fry	Pork Chops with Fennel, Onion and Pears with Crispy Carrots and Garlic	Honey-Garlic Chicken with Garlic and Chive Butter Brussels Sprouts	Sesame-Ginger Chicken Tacos in Jicama Shells

	DAY 7	DAY 8	DAY 9	DAY 10	DAY 11	DAY 12
BREAKFAST	Overnight Cherry-Chia Smoothie	Apple and Carrot Muffins	"PB and J" Chia Pudding	Spiced-Up Eggs Over Greens	Creamy Mango Smoothie	Kale and Sweet Potato Egg Muffins
LUNCH	Thyme and Oregano Turkey Burger with Crispy Carrots and Garlic	Sweet and Savory Chicken Salad Wrap with Garlic and Chive Butter Brussels Sprouts	Chicken and Sage "Noodle" Soup with optional slice of Rosemary and Salt Bread	Chicken and Pesto Collard Wrap with Sweet Potato Latkes	Chicken Sausage, Kale and Sweet Potato Soup with optional slice of Rosemary and Salt Bread	Apple, Pecan and Chicken Arugula Salad
DINNER	Lamb Lollipops with Basil and Pea Puree with Sweet Potato Latkes	Chicken, Sweet Potato, Apple and Broccoli Skillet	Kale Pesto Cheesy Chicken with Caramelized Fennel	Beef and Cabbage Hash with Mashed Japanese Sweet Potatoes	Poached Chicken and Green Beans in Ginger Broth	Pork Medallions with Shaved Brussels and Carrots

	DAY 13	DAY 14	DAY 15	DAY 16	DAY 17	DAY 18
BREAKFAST	Apple Bread	Asparagus and Red Potato Frittata	Overnight Cherry-Chia Smoothie	Apple and Carrot Muffins	"PB and J" Chia Pudding	Spiced-Up Eggs Over Greens
LUNCH	Rosemary and Garlic Lamb Burger with Caramelized Fennel	Kale and Onion Chicken Patty Wrap with Mashed Japanese Sweet Potatoes	Artichoke Soup with optional slice of Rosemary and Salt Bread	Chicken and Mango Salad	Thyme and Oregano Turkey Burger with Crispy Carrots and Garlic	Sweet and Savory Chicken Salad Wrap with Garlic and Chive Butter Brussels Sprouts
DINNER	Instant Pot Chicken with Gravy and Cauliflower Mash	Antihistamine Chicken Stir-Fry	Pork Chops with Fennel, Onion and Pears with Crispy Carrots and Garlic	Honey-Garlic Chicken with Garlic and Chive Butter Brussels Sprouts	Sesame-Ginger Chicken Tacos in Jicama Shells	Lamb Lollipops with Basil and Pea Puree with Sweet Potato Latkes

	DAY 19	DAY 20	DAY 21	DAY 22	DAY 23	DAY 24
BREAKFAST	Creamy Mango Smoothie	Kale and Sweet Potato Egg Muffins	Apple Bread	Asparagus and Red Potato Frittata	Overnight Cherry-Chia Smoothie	Apple and Carrot Muffins
LUNCH	Chicken and Sage "Noodle" Soup with optional slice of Rosemary and Salt Bread	Chicken and Pesto Collard Wrap with Sweet Potato Latkes	Chicken Sausage, Kale and Sweet Potato Soup with optional slice of Rosemary and Salt Bread	Apple, Pecan and Chicken Arugula Salad	Rosemary and Garlic Lamb Burger with Caramelized Fennel	Kale and Onion Chicken Patty Wrap with Mashed Japanese Sweet Potatoes
DINNER	Chicken, Sweet Potato, Apple and Broccoli Skillet	Kale Pesto Cheesy Chicken with Caramelized Fennel	Beef and Cabbage Hash with Mashed Japanese Sweet Potatoes	Poached Chicken and Green Beans in Ginger Broth	Pork Medallions with Shaved Brussels and Carrots	Instant Pot Chicken with Gravy and Cauliflower Mash

	DAY 25	DAY 26	DAY 27	DAY 28	DAY 29	DAY 30
BREAKFAST	"PB and J" Chia Pudding	Spiced-Up Eggs Over Greens	Creamy Mango Smoothie	Kale and Sweet Potato Egg Muffins	Creamy Mango Smoothie	Kale and Sweet Potato Egg Muffins
LUNCH	Artichoke Soup with optional slice of Rosemary and Salt Bread	Chicken and Mango Salad	Thyme and Oregano Turkey Burger with Crispy Carrots and Garlic	Sweet and Savory Chicken Salad Wrap with Garlic and Chive Butter Brussels Sprouts	Chicken and Sage "Noodle" Soup with optional slice of Rosemary and Salt Bread	Chicken and Pesto Collard Wrap with Sweet Potato Latkes
DINNER	Antihistamine Chicken Stir-Fry	Pork Chops with Fennel, Onion and Pears with Crispy Carrots and Garlic	Honey-Garlic Chicken with Garlic and Chive Butter Brussels Sprouts	Sesame-Ginger Chicken Tacos in Jicama Shells	Lamb Lollipops with Basil and Pea Puree with Sweet Potato Latkes	Chicken, Sweet Potato, Apple and Broccoli Skillet

ADDITIONAL **RESOURCES**

SUPPLEMENTS FOR HISTAMINE INTOLERANCE

There are countless supplements available now, and some may be helpful for histamine intolerance while others, not so much.

For this reason, it is important to be careful with supplements. Probiotics, for example, which are generally considered safe and healthy, may actually cause a histamine issue in those with histamine intolerance.

Here's a breakdown of the supplements I recommend and those I advise staying away from.

RECOMMENDED SUPPLEMENTS

Vitamin C

Vitamin C is a great supplement for supporting immune health, but it also works as a natural antihistamine. You will want to choose a vitamin C supplement that is made from ascorbyl palmitate and avoid the most commonly seen vitamin C supplement available, ascorbic acid. This form usually comes from corn, which is not something we want to be eating on the low-histamine diet, as many people are allergic to it.

DAO

DAO is one of the most talked about supplements when it comes to histamine intolerance because it is an enzyme present in the body that helps break down histamine. However, for those with histamine intolerance, there may not be enough DAO present to break down the histamine, leading to a buildup.

For those who don't have enough of this enzyme present in their body, taking a DAO supplement may be necessary. Supplementing with DAO may not be necessary forever, as once the histamine intolerance is under control, the body may be able to start creating adequate amounts of DAO. However, some people are born without enough DAO, and supplementation may be needed long term. As with anything else, this is going to vary from person to person.

DAO supplements are typically taken when you have consumed food or drink high in histamines, and should not be taken daily if following the diet. Seeking Health makes a great DAO supplement called Histamine Block.

Quercetin

Quercetin is one of the most recommended supplements when it comes to histamine intolerance. Quercetin works by directly blocking the release of histamine from the mast cells. Quercetin also has anti-inflammatory and antiviral properties, which can work well when dealing with the root causes of histamine intolerance. See page 60 for foods high in quercetin.

Stinging Nettles (Nettle Extract)

Stinging nettles, or *Urtica dioica*, is a plant that can reduce the amount of histamine the body produces. It has been shown to be as effective as antihistamine medication like Claritin, Zyrtec and others without reducing DAO enzyme activity in the body.

Selenium

Selenium is a nutrient found in foods like Brazil nuts, organ meats, eggs and more. Selenium is a powerful nutrient with many health benefits, including supporting the thyroid gland. What many don't know about selenium is that it is also important for reducing mast cell activation. This makes selenium a very important nutrient to those suffering with histamine intolerance.

The next section is going to give you my exact plan for supporting histamine intolerance using a few vital supplements. This plan is a good overall base for those suffering with histamine intolerance that most can easily tolerate. Some may require a more specific plan based on their underlying cause (or causes) of histamine intolerance, but this is a good place to start.

DR. BECKY'S FAVORITE STORE-BOUGHT ITEMS

One of the hardest things about following a low-histamine food plan is that everything needs to be made fresh. Although this is true for most food items, I have put together a list of prepackaged foods you can safely consume that should not adversely affect the way you feel (see page 177).

While I recommend making as much as you can, especially during the initial phase of elimination, it's also okay to pick up some Paleo-friendly things at the store (especially once you have your symptoms firmly under control).

Thrive Market
https://thrivemarket.com

Thrive Market, an online wholesale store, offers abundant, affordable healthy foods that you can order and have delivered straight to your door! I highly recommend this site to anyone who is looking to save some money or doesn't have a health food store local to them, as Thrive Market offers just about any healthy grab-and-go option.

DR. BECKY'S HISTAMINE INTOLERANCE SUPPLEMENT PLAN

HISTO RELIEF

This is my favorite supplement to support histamine intolerance or MCAS. Histo Relief is a mast cell stabilizing supplement that supports immune function as well as the body's response to food and environmental factors. It aids in gastrointestinal function and antioxidant processes.

Histo Relief is a blend of nutrients like quercetin, nettle leaf and vitamin C, which can be very helpful in stabilizing mast cells. It also contains Tinofend, extracted from the plant *Tinospora cordifolia*, which has been shown to regulate key immune mediators and support activity of the macrophages. This supports the immune response by promoting balance of phagocytic white blood cells and eosinophils. It does an excellent job supporting those with histamine intolerance and MCAS. This supplement also contains quercetin, which helps stabilize mast cells. Many people use it as a natural way to help control allergy symptoms.

ULTIMATE GUT SUPPORT

Supporting the integrity of the gut lining is crucial when working with histamine intolerance. The lining of the gut must have the proper permeability and integrity so it can prevent allergens, microbes and toxins from gaining access to the bloodstream. Since leaky gut is one of the biggest triggers for histamine intolerance, this supplement can be extremely helpful when you're trying to tolerate more foods.

PROBIOTICS

The topic of probiotics always comes up when I'm talking to my clients about supplements. Many people use them as a way to support healthy gut flora, which is essential to proper digestive function and overall health. However, probiotics are not the best option for those with histamine intolerance because they are fermented.

The tricky thing here is that you need healthy digestive function for the enzymes DAO and monoamine oxidase to work as they should. However, we need to be careful about what supplement we choose. Not only are most probiotic supplements fermented, but some strains of beneficial bacteria can raise histamine. The good news is that there are some strains that have been shown to lower histamine.

With limited research on histamine intolerance and probiotics, the following strains have been found to be acceptable for those with histamine intolerance and they may also be able to reduce inflammation:

- *Bifidobacterium bifidum*
- *Bifidobacterium infantis*
- *Bifidobacterium longum*
- *Bifidobacterium lactis*
- *Lactobacillus rhamnosus*
- *Lactobacillus plantarum*
- *Lactobacillus salivarius*

The company Seeking Health makes a probiotic called ProBiota HistaminX that has all but one of these strains of bacteria.

PROBIOTICS TO AVOID

Some species of bacteria that should be avoided with histamine intolerance include the following:

- *Lactobacillus bulgaricus*
- *Lactobacillus casei*
- *Lactobacillus delbrueckii*
- *Lactobacillus helveticus*
- *Streptococcus thermophilus*

DIGEST CARE

As we talked about earlier, digestive enzymes are extremely important for those suffering with histamine intolerance. Since most people with histamine intolerance have some type of issue with their gut health (i.e., SIBO or leaky gut), they tend to need more help breaking down food properly. The Digest Care supplement can be found at https://shop-dr-becky-campbell.myshopify.com.

LIVER LOVE

While methods like infrared saunas, Epsom salt baths and other natural liver support methods we talked about earlier can be very effective, they can also be very time-consuming. The Optimal Reset Liver Love supplement (found on my website) contains nutrients like milk thistle and NAC (a derivative of the amino acid cysteine, which has powerful antioxidant and liver-protective actions). In addition to protecting the body from oxidative stress, NAC assists with the formation of glutathione, the predominant antioxidant found in the liver, and is shown to have an inhibitory effect on mast cells.

SUPPLEMENTATION SCHEDULE

Here is how I recommend taking the preceding supplements:

- Histo Relief: 2 capsules twice per day
- Optimal Reset Liver Love: 2 capsules twice per day
- Digest Care: 2 capsules per meal
- Ultimate Gut Support: 1 scoop twice per day on an empty stomach (mix with water)

The preceding supplements can be found on my website: www.DrBeckyCampbell.com.

Here is how I recommend taking the Seeking Health supplements:

- Seeking Health ProBiota HistaminX: 1 capsule twice per day
- Seeking Health Histamine Block: Can be taken with food or drinks that contain high levels of histamine (perfect if you are having wine)

The preceding supplements can be found at www.seekinghealth.com.

FAVORITE PACKAGED AND PREPARED FOODS

Siete Brand
https://sietefoods.com

YES

Cassava and coconut tortilla shells; cassava and chia tortilla shells

MAYBE

Almond flour tortilla shells

NO

Any of their products containing avocado oil (like their tortilla chips), tortilla shells containing cashews or chickpeas, hot sauces

Simple Mills
https://www.simplemills.com

MAYBE

Their rosemary and sea salt crackers, artisan bread mix, pizza dough mix, vanilla cake mix, pecan cookies (if you do well with almond flour)

NO

Products containing chocolate, tomato, banana, cheddar, cinnamon and peanut butter

Legit Bread Company
http://www.legitbreadcompany.com

This is one of my favorite brands to make life easier with histamine intolerance. I use their bread mixes regularly in my house and they make food prep quick and easy. The only thing you could possibly have a problem with is apple cider vinegar, which is one of the lowest-histamine vinegars. I have actually made these bread mixes without the apple cider vinegar and they come out just fine.

YES

Bagel mix, sandwich bread mix, pancake mix

NUCO
https://shop.nucoconut.com/

I eat their wraps almost every day. I find them extremely convenient and they taste amazing!

YES

Coconut wraps, original and garlic coconut oil

MAYBE

Coconut Crunch cereal, lemon herb coconut oil

NO

Coconut vinegars (fermented)

SPICES

When using dried spices, make sure to stay away from ones listed on the No List (like cinnamon, anise, curry powder, hot paprika and nutmeg). There are two brands of spices that I love and trust:

Primal Palate Organic
https://www.primalpalate.com/organic-spices

I love every one of their spices and trust that they are coming from a good source.

Balanced Bites Spices
https://shop.balancedbites.com/collections/spices

They have an amazing bagel spice that goes great with the Legit Bread brand bagel mix.

TRACKING TOOLS

I love tracking tools because they are an excellent way to help pinpoint certain dietary and lifestyle choices that may be making your symptoms worse. Here are some of my favorite tracking tools:

- mySymptoms Food Diary: available on iTunes for iOs devices.

This app offers reviews and comments on 700 different foods.

- Food Intolerances: http://www.baliza.de/en/apps/histamine.html

STRESS MANAGEMENT

With histamine intolerance, it is important to manage your stress levels, because as we've seen, high levels of stress can be a triggering factor. Simple practices like meditation and visualization techniques can help lower your stress levels substantially. You are not alone if you think that meditation is not for you, that there is no way it could change your life. But consider the following: Studies show that meditation can actually change the structure and function of your brain permanently.

Try the exercise on page 180 for 30 consecutive days. Find a quiet spot for 10 minutes in the morning and listen to a guided meditation track via a meditation app or other platform.

Then do the same during the afternoon or early evening, this time guiding yourself through a positive visualization.

FAQS

1. HOW DOES HISTAMINE AFFECT THE BRAIN?

Histamine intolerance may affect brain health more than you think. It has actually been linked to Tourette's syndrome, a condition characterized by tics, which take the form of involuntary movements and vocalizations. Nearly half of those that suffer from this condition also have an accompanying condition, such as ADHD or OCD.

Tourette's syndrome is thought to have a genetic link. A study published in the *New England Journal of Medicine* by Matthew State, MD, PhD, has linked a gene mutation to Tourette's syndrome. The study looked at a family in which the father had Tourette's and OCD, all eight children had Tourette's and two of them also had OCD. Dr. State determined that all of the family members suffering from these conditions had a histidine decarboxylase (HDC) gene mutation. This gene is required to encode an enzyme needed for histamine production. When the HDC mutation is present, it reduces the activity of this specific enzyme.

Keep in mind that not everyone with this gene mutation will have Tourette's syndrome. In fact, the researchers did not find the mutation in 700 other people who had Tourette's syndrome. However, the study is very interesting due to the fact it may show how histamine functions in the brain.

Studies have also found that mice that do not have the HDC gene are also prone to having repetitive behaviors, similar to the tics that occur in Tourette's syndrome. These mice were found to improve once they were given medications that act on histamine receptors in the brain. Histamine and dopamine also interact, and dopamine happens to be commonly used in drugs to help reduce Tourette's symptoms.

The more researchers look into Tourette's syndrome, the more it appears that histamine may play a fairly significant role in Tourette's syndrome. The family that was being studied is still involved in research to determine histamine's role in Tourette's syndrome, and further genetic research into the condition continues to move forward.

High levels of histamine in the brain have also been shown to cause issues with the release of certain neurotransmitters like serotonin, dopamine and norepinephrine. When histamine levels are too high, things like overstimulation can occur, making you feel off balance.

2. IS THERE A CONNECTION BETWEEN DEPRESSION AND HISTAMINE INTOLERANCE?

Yes. When histamine levels are elevated in the body, it can lead to depression and even OCD. When there is an alteration in any biochemistry, it can cause mental health changes. Working to get your histamine levels under control may help you feel better both physically and mentally.

3. ARE THERE DOCTORS WHO SPECIALIZE IN MAST CELL ACTIVATION SYNDROME?

Yes. Here are the practitioners I recommend:

- Dr. Jill Carnahan:
  https://www.jillcarnahan.com/
- Dr. Lawrence B. Afrin:
  http://mastcellresearch.com/
- Dr. T. C. Theoharides:
   http://www.mastcellmaster.com/

VISUALIZATION EXERCISE TO REDUCE FOOD REACTIONS

1. Find a comfortable position, sitting in a chair or lying on your back. Rest your hands at your sides and close your eyes.

2. Take a deep breath, letting the air out with a sigh. Let your body fully relax and feel the stress slip away as you breathe.

3. Focus on how your body feels right now, noticing where your body is tense, and relax those areas with each breath.

4. Then tense up your muscles in those areas for a few seconds. Hold and relax. Repeat this process a few times.

5. If you feel fear of any kind, choose to now calmly acknowledge that fear, and be kind and supportive of yourself as you observe your fear. Know that you are getting through the discomfort, feeling better and calmer with every passing moment.

6. Allow your mind to become calm and relaxed. Feel everything settling down. Your mind, body and spirit can relax.

7. Now focus on visualizing your body happily receiving nourishment. Feel the goodness that comes from your diet, vitamins, minerals and energy. Let the pleasant feelings wash over you.

8. After a few minutes, or as long as you would like, wiggle your fingers and toes to wake up your limbs. Stretch if you want to. Open your eyes.

9. Take a moment to sit quietly and reorient to your surroundings, then go about your normal activities.

For best results, make a few notes on how you feel at the beginning of the 30-day period. Are you stressed? If so, how stressed are you on a scale of 1 to 10? Do the exercise again at the end of the experiment. You will be amazed at the results, and I can guarantee that you will be happy with the physical improvements you feel too.

REFERENCES

CHAPTER 1

Ballantyne, S. (The Paleo Mom). "Did you know that histamine intolerance might mean your thyroid is out of whack? Both hypothyroidism and hyperthyroidism affect histamine." Facebook post, February 19, 2014. https://www.facebook.com/thepaleomom/posts/did-you-know-that-histamine-intolerance-might-mean-your-thyroid-is-out-of-whack-/828092583881939.

Chikahisa, S., T. Kodama, A. Soya, Y. Sagawa, Y. Ishimaru, H. Séi and S. Nishino. "Histamine from Brain Resident MAST Cells Promotes Wakefulness and Modulates Behavioral States." *PLoS One* 8, no. 10 (October 2018). https://doi.org/10.1371/journal.pone.0078434.

Christ, P., A. S. Sowa, O. Froy and A. Lorentz. "The Circadian Clock Drives Mast Cell Functions in Allergic Reactions." *Frontiers in Immunology* 9, article 1526 (July 2018). https://doi.org/10.3389/fimmu.2018.01526.

Davidson, R. J., and A. Lutz. "Buddha's Brain: Neuroplasticity and Meditation." *IEEE Signal Processing Magazine* 25, no. 1 (January 2008): 174–176. https://www.ncbi.nlm.nih.gov/pmc/articles/PMC2944261.

"HER-stamine? The Link Between Histamine and Estrogen." MTHFR Support Australia. https://www.mthfrsupport.com.au/her-stamine-the-link-between-histamine-and-estrogen.

"Immunoglobulin E (IgE) Definition." American Academy of Allergy Asthma and Immunology. https://www.aaaai.org/conditions-and-treatments/conditions-dictionary/immunoglobulin-e-(ige).

Jockers, D. "Are You Suffering from Histamine Intolerance?" DrJockers.com. https://drjockers.com/suffering histamine-intolerance.

Kresser, C. "RHR: What You Should Know about Histamine Intolerance." Chris Kresser. November 28, 2014. https://chriskresser.com/what-you-should-know-about-histamine-intolerance.

Lam, M., and J. Lam. "Histamine Levels and Adrenal Fatigue Syndrome—Part 2." Dr. Lam Coaching. https://www.drlam.com/blog/histamine-levels/5906.

Maintz, L., and N. Novak. "Histamine and Histamine Intolerance." *American Journal of Clinical Nutrition* 85, no. 1 (May 2007): 1185–1196. https://doi.org/10.1093/ajcn/85.5.1185.

Meskanen, K., H. Ekelund, J. Laitinen, P. J. Neuvonen, J. Haukka, P. Panula and J. Ekelund. "A Randomized Clinical Trial of Histamine 2 Receptor Antagonism in Treatment-Resistant Schizophrenia." *Journal of Clinical Psychopharmacology* 33, no. 4 (August 2013): 472–478. https://www.ncbi.nlm.nih.govpubmed/23764683.

Muñoz-Cruz, S., Y. Mendoza-Rodríguez, K. E. Nava-Castro, L. Yepez-Mulia and J. Morales-Montor. "Gender-Related Effects of Sex Steroids on Histamine Release and FcεRI Expression in Rat Peritoneal Mast Cells." *Journal of Immunology Research*, article ID 351829 (February 2015): 10 pages. http://dx.doi.org/10.1155/2015/351829.

Myers, A. "Everything You Need to Know about Histamine Intolerance." Amy Myers MD. https://www.amymyersmd.com/2017/10/everything-you-need-to-know-about- histamine-intolerance.

Nautiyal, K. M., A. C. Ribeiro, D. W. Pfaff and R. Silver. "Brain Mast Cells Link the Immune System to Anxiety-Like Behavior." *Proceedings of the National Academy of Sciences of the United States of America* 105, no. 46 (November 2008): 18053–18057. https://doi.org/10.1073/pnas.0809479105.

"Relaxation for Dealing with Food Sensitivities." Inner Health Studio. https://www.innerhealthstudio.com/food-sensitivities.html.

Schneider. E., M. Leite-de-moraes and M. Dy. "Histamine, Immune Cells and Autoimmunity." *Advances in Experimental Medicine and Biology* 709 (2010): 81–94. https://www.ncbi.nlm.nih.gov/pubmed/21618890.

Weinshilboum, R. M., D. M. Otterness and C. L. Szumlanski. "Methylation Pharmacogenetics Catechol-O Methyltransferase Thiopurine Methyltransferase, and Histamine N-Methyltransferase." *Annual Review of Pharmacology and Toxicology* 19 (April 1999): 19–52. https://doi.org/10.1146/annurev.pharmtox.39.1.19.

"What Are Histamines?" WebMD. https://www.webmd.com/allergies/what-are-histamines#1.

Zierau, O., A. C. Zenclussen and F. Jensen. "Role of Female Sex Hormones, Estradiol and Progesterone, in Mast Cell Behavior." *Frontiers in Immunology* 3, article 169 (June 2012). https://doi.org/10.3389/fimmu.2012.00169.

CHAPTER 2

Afrin, L. B., S. Self, J. Menk and J. Lazarchick. "Characterization of Mast Cell Activation Syndrome." *American Journal of the Medical Sciences* 353, no. 3 (March 2017): 207–215. https://doi.org/10.1016/j.amjms.2016.12.013.

Alexander, A. "Mast Cell Activation Disease vs. Histamine Intolerance (Differences)." Alvin Alexander (blog). Updated February 6, 2019. https://alvinalexander.com/personal/differences-mast-cell-activation-disease-vs-histamine-intolerance.

Alexander, B. J., B. N. Ames, S. M. Baker and P. Bennet. *Textbook of Functional Medicine.* Edited by D. S. Jones and S. Quinn. Washington, DC: The Institute for Functional Medicine, 2010: 3–66.

Atherton, J. C., and M. J. Blaser. "Coadaptation of *Helicobacter pylori* and Humans: Ancient History, Modern Implications." *Journal of Clinical Investigation* 119, no. 9 (September 2009): 2475–2487. https://doi.org/10.1172 JCI38605.

Axe, J. "9 Candida Symptoms and 3 Steps to Treat Them." Dr. Axe. January 26, 2019. https://draxe.com/candida-symptoms.

Basso D., F. Navaglia, L. Brigato, F. Di Mario, M. Rugge and M. Plebani. "*Helicobacter pylori* Non-Cytotoxic Genotype Enhances Mucosal Gastrin and Mast Cell Tryptase." *Journal of Clinical Pathology* 52 (March 1999): 210–214. https://jcp.bmj.com/content/jclinpath/52/3/210.full.pdf.

Buric, I., M. Farias, J. Jong, C. Mee and I. A. Brazil. "What Is the Molecular Signature of Mind-Body Interventions? A Systematic Review of Gene Expression Changes Induced by Meditation and Related Practices." *Frontiers in Immunology* 8, article 670 (June 2017). https://doi.org/10.3389/fimmu.2017.00670.

Burkhart, A. "Histamine Intolerance: Could It Be Causing Your Symptoms?" Amy Burkhart, MD. http://theceliacmd.com/2014/03/histamine-intolerance-causing-symptoms.

"Diagnosis and Treatment of MCAS (Mast Cell Activation Syndrome)." InHealth RVA. April 17, 2018. https://www.integrativehealthrichmond.org/single-post/2018/04/17/Diagnosis-and-Treatment-of-MCAS-Mast-Cell-Activation-Syndrome-aka-everything-I-take-do-or-am-exposed-to-makes-me-feel-horrible.

Figura, N., A. Perrone, C. Gennari, G. Orlandini, L. Bianciardi, R. Giannace et al. "Food Allergy and *Helicobacter pylori* Infection." *Italian Journal of Gastroenterology and Hepatology* 31, no. 3 (April 1999): 186–191. https://www.ncbi.nlm.nih.gov/pubmed/10379477.

Guthrie, C. "How to Heal a Leaky Gut." *Experience Life* magazine. March 2015. https://experiencelife.com/article/how-to-heal-a-leaky-gut.

"*Helicobacter pylori* (*H. pylori*) Infection." Mayo Clinic. May 17, 2017. https://www.mayoclinic.org/diseases-conditions/h-pylori/symptoms-causes/syc-20356171.

Joneja, J. "Histamine and Mast Cell Activation Disorder." Foods Matter. https://www.histamine-sensitivity.com/histamine-mastocytosis-joneja-05-15.html.

Kihara, T., S. Biro, Y. Ikeda, T. Fukudome, T. Shinsato, A. Masuda et al. "Effects of Repeated Sauna Treatment on Ventricular Arrhythmias in Patients with Chronic Heart Failure." *Circulation Journal* 68, no. 12 (December 2004): 1146–1151. https://www.ncbi.nlm.nih.gov/pubmed/15564698.

Kresser, C. "RHR: Candida—Hidden Epidemic or Fad Diagnosis?" Chris Kresser. September 26, 2017. https://chriskresser.com/candida-hidden-epidemic-or-fad-diagnosis.

———. "RHR: How to Tell If You Have a Leaky Gut." Chris Kresser. September 1, 2016. https://chriskresser.com/how-to-tell-if-you-have-a-leaky-gut.

———. "Still Think Gluten Sensitivity Isn't Real?" Chris Kresser. August 23, 2016. https://chriskresser.com/still-think-gluten-sensitivity-isnt-real.

Lunger, C. "The Real Truth about *H. pylori*: Allergies, Autoimmune, and Adrenal Fatigue." Gutsy (blog). May 5, 2013. http://www.mygutsy.com/is-h-pylori-the-cause-of-allergies-brain-fog-hypothyroid-autoimmune-disorders-adrenal-fatigue.

Lynch, B. "Does SIBO Affect Histamine Intolerance and DAO?" Dr. Ben Lynch. https://www.drbenlynch.com/sibo-histamine.

———. "Histamine Intolerance, MTHFR and Methylation." MTHRF.net. June 11, 2015. http://mthfr.net/histamine-intolerance-mthfr-and methylation/2015/06/11.

Ma, Z. F., N. A. Majid, Y. Yamaoka and Y. Y. Lee. "Food Allergy and *Helicobacter pylori* Infection: A Systematic Review." *Frontiers in Microbiology* 7, article 368 (March 2016). https://doi.org/10.3389/fmicb.2016.00368.

Malfertheiner, P., F. Megraud, C. A. O'Morain, J. P. Gisbert, E. J. Kuipers, A. T. Axon et al. "Management of *Helicobacter pylori* Infection—The Maastricht V/Florence Consensus Report." *Gut* 66 (2017): 6–30. https://www.ncbi.nlm.nih.gov/pubmed/27707777.

Masuda, A., Y. Koga, M. Hattanmaru, S. Minagoe and C. Tei. "The Effects of Repeated Thermal Therapy for Patients with Chronic Pain." *Psychotherapy and Psychosomatics* 74, no. 5 (2005): 288–294. https://doi.org/10.1159/000086319.

Mercola, J. "17 Micrograms of Lead in Your Body Lowers Your IQ by 10 Points." Mercola. March 21, 2012. https://articles.mercola.com/sites/articles/archive/2012/03/21/dr-clement-on-detoxification.aspx.

Merizalde, K. "Histamine Intolerance and Its Relationship to Minerals." Sassy Holistics. March 24, 2016. https://www.sassyholistics.com/2016/03/24/histamine-intolerance.

Sears, M. E., K. J. Kerr, and R. I. Bray. "Arsenic, Cadmium, Lead, and Mercury in Sweat: A Systematic Review." *Journal of Environmental and Public Health* 2012, article ID 184745 (February 2012): 10 pages. http://dx.doi.org/10.1155/2012/184745.

Seneviratne, S. L., A. Maitland and L. Afrin. "Mast Cell Disorders in Ehlers-Danlos Syndrome." *American Journal of Medical Genetics Part C: Seminars in Medical Genetics* 175, no. 1 (March 2017): 226–236. https://doi.org/10.1002/ajmg.c.31555.

"Systemic Mastocytosis." National Center for Advancing Translational Sciences, Genetic and Rare Diseases Information Center. https://rarediseases.info.nih.gov/diseases/8616/systemic-mastocytosis.

"Ulcerative Colitis." Mayo Clinic. March 8, 2018. https://www.mayoclinic.org/diseases-conditions/ulcerative-colitis/symptoms-causes/syc-20353326.

"What Is Crohn's Disease?" Crohn's and Colitis Foundation. http://www.crohnscolitisfoundation.org/what-are-crohns-and-colitis/what-is-crohns-disease.

Ykelenstam, Y. "Are You Allergic to Candida?" Healing Histamine. https://healinghistamine.com/are-you-allergic-to-candida.

CHAPTER 3

"Cleaning Supplies and Household Chemicals." American Lung Association. http://www.lung.org/our-initiatives/healthy-air/indoor/indoor-air-pollutants/cleaning-supplies-household-chem.html.

Larsen, B. "Allergies and the Bucket Theory of Toxicity." Dr. Brant Larsen. http://drlarsen.com/allergies-and-the-bucket-theory-of-toxicity.

CHAPTER 4

"Food Compatibility List." Swiss Interest Group Histamine Intolerance. https://www.mastzellaktivierung.info/downloads/foodlist/21_FoodList_EN_alphabetic_withCateg.pdf.

Levy, J. "Quercetin: 8 Proven Benefits of This Antioxidant (#1 Is Incredible)." Dr. Axe. October 2, 2018. https://draxe.com/quercetin.

"SIGHI-Leaflet Histamine Elimination Diet: Simplified Histamine Elimination Diet for Histamine Intolerance (DAO Degradation Disorder)." Swiss Interest Group Histamine Intolerance (SIGHI). July 7, 2017. https://www.histaminintoleranz.ch/downloads/SIGHI-Leaflet_HistamineEliminationDiet.pdf.

Ykelenstam, Y. "How to Naturally Boost Production of the Histamine Degrading DAO Enzyme." Healing Histamine. https://healinghistamine.com/how-to-naturally-boost-production-of-the-histamine-degrading-dao-enzyme.

CHAPTER 5

"5 Health Benefits of Cauliflower." P. Allen Smith Garden Home. September 13, 2017. https://pallensmith.com/2017/09/13/health-benefits-cauliflower.

"16 Natural Antihistamine Foods (Plus Benefits!)" Prana Thrive. https://pranathrive.com/natural-antihistamine-foods.

Banerjee, M., and P. K. Sarkar. "Inhibitory Effect of Garlic on Bacterial Pathogens from Spices." *World Journal of Microbiology and Biotechnology* 19, no. 6 (August 2003): 565–569. https://doi.org/10.1023/A:1025108116389.

Barrington, R. "Cabbage, Glutamine and the Gut." RdB Nutrition (blog). May 2, 2015. http://www.robertbarington.net/cabbage-glutamine-gut/.

"Cassava: Benefits and Dangers." Healthline. March 24, 2017. https://www.healthline.com/nutritioncassava#section1.

Cownley, S. "Top 20 Antihistamine Foods That Help Fight Inflammation." Foods for Better Health. https://www.foodsforbetterhealth.com/top-20-antihistamine-foods-that-help-fight-inflammation-28555.

Donelson, H. "Antihistamine Juice." Happy Tummies Digestive Health and Nutrition Balancing. March 23, 2016. https://happytummiesdigest.com/2016/03/23/antihistamine-juice.

Forberg, C. "5 Powerful Health Benefits of Asparagus You Probably Didn't Know." *EatingWell*. http://www.eatingwell.com/article/17129/5-powerful-health-benefits-of-asparagus-you-probably-didnt-know.

Hensley, L. "Tiger Nuts: What Are They, and Are They Good for You?" Global News. September 25, 2018. https://globalnews.ca/news/4480574/tiger-nuts.

Jockers, D. "Are You Suffering from Histamine Intolerance?" DrJockers.com. https://drjockers.com/suffering-histamine-intolerance.

Julia, Fp. "The Benefits of Purple Foods." BLDG 25. March 14, 2013. https://blog.freepeople.com/2013/03/benefits-purple-foods.

Link, R. "8 Surprising Health Benefits of Cloves." Healthline. August 26, 2017. https://www.healthline.com/nutrition/benefits-of-cloves#section5.

Link, R. "Chia Seeds Benefits: The Omega-3, Protein-Packed Superfood." Dr. Axe. January 24, 2019. https://draxe.com/chia-seeds-benefits-side-effects.

Link, R. "Top 7 Benefits of Blueberries." Dr. Axe. April 30, 2018. https://draxe.com/health-benefits-blueberries.

Philpott, V. "Are There Foods That Act as Antihistamines?" LIVESTRONG. https://www.livestrong.com/article/134112-foods-that-act-as-antihistamine.

"Quercetin, A Natural Antihistamine." BioXtract. http://www.bioxtract.com/plant-based-actives/quercetin/index.html.

Scully, E. "Histamine and Anti-Histamine Foods." A Lust for Life. https://www.alustforlife.com/physical-health/nutrition-physical-health/histamine-and-anti-histamine-foods.

Sivaram, S. "Reasons Why You Should Never Eat Corn Again." Boldsky. January 30, 2017. https://www.boldsky.com/health/wellness/2017/reasons-why-you-should-never-eat-corn-again/articlecontent-pf145886-110563.html.

Vickery, A. "21 Anti-Histamine Foods That Fight Inflammation and Stabilise Mast-Cells." Alison Vickery. September 23, 2014. http://alisonvickery.com.au/anti-histamine-foods.

Ware, M. "What Are the Benefits of Chia Seeds?" Medical News Today. Updated November 12, 2018. https://www.medicalnewstoday.com/articles/291334.php.

——. "Why Is Fennel Good for You?" Medical News Today. Updated August 23, 2018. https://www.medicalnewstoday.com/articles/284096.php.

"What Is Jicama (Yambean) Good For?" Food Facts Presented by Mercola. October 25, 2016. https://foodfacts.mercola.com/jicama.html.

Ykelenstam, Y. "7 Best Foods for Histamine Intolerance." Healing Histamine. https://healinghistamine.com/7-best-foods-for-histamine-intolerance.

APPENDIX

Bryan, L. "5 Things You Need to Know About Cassava Flour." Downshiftology. July 7, 2017. https://downshiftology.com/5-things-you-need-to-know-about-cassava-flour.

Carnahan, J. "Mast Cell Activation Syndrome (MCAS): When Histamine Goes Haywire." Dr. Jill. October 31, 2016. https://www.jillcarnahan.com/2016/10/31/mast-cell-activation-syndrome-mcas-when-histamine-goes-haywire.

——. "Mold Is a Major Trigger of Mast Activation Cell Syndrome." Dr. Jill. March 12, 2018. https://www.jillcarnahan.com/2018/03/12/mold-is-a-major-trigger-of-mast-activation-cell-syndrome.

Ferreria, C. G. T., M. G. Campos, D. M. Felix, M. R. Santos, O. V. de Carvalho, M. A. N. Diaz et al. "Evaluation of the Antiviral Activities of *Bacharis dracunculifolia* and Quercetin on *Equid herpesvirus 1* in a Murine Model." *Research in Veterinary Science* 120 (October 2018): 70–77. https://doi.org/10.1016/j.rvsc.2018.09.001.

Harris, J. "What Is Tigernut Flour?" *Gluten-Free Living*. September 3, 2015. https://www.glutenfreeliving.com/blog/what-is-tigernut-flour.

McGruther, J. "Coconut Flour: Baking Tips, Substitutions and Recipes." Nourished Kitchen (blog). https://nourishedkitchen.com/baking-with-coconut-flour.

Price, A. "Coconut Flour Nutrition: The Gluten-Free Flour Substitute That Boosts Health." Dr. Axe. February 5, 2019. https://draxe.com/coconut-flour-nutrition.

Rahm, D. H. "Bromelain and Quercetin: Balance the Natural Inflammatory Response." VitaMedica. December 4, 2012. https://vitamedica.com/wellness-blog/bromelain-and-quercetin-natural-anti-inflammatory-supplements.

Roscheck Jr., B., R. C. Fink, M. McMichael and R. S. Alberte. "Nettle Extract (*Urtica dioica*) Affects Key Receptors and Enzymes Associated with Allergic Rhinitis." *Phytotherapy Research* 23, no. 7 (July 2009): 920–926. https://doi.org/10.1002/ptr.2763.

Safaralizadeh, R., M. Nourizadeh, A. Zare, G. A. Kardar and Z. Pourpak. "Influence of Selenium on Mast Cell Mediator Release." *Biological Trace Element Research* 154, no. 2 (August 2013): 299–303. https://doi.org/10.1007/s12011-013-9712-x.

"The Ultimate Guide to Coconut Flour vs Almond Flour." Ditch the Carbs. https://www.ditchthecarbs.com/ultimate-guide-coconut-flour-vs-almond-flour.

Ykelenstam, Y. "Parasites Trigger Mast Cell Histamine Release." Healing Histamine. https://healinghistamine.com/parasites-trigger-mast-cell-histamine-release.

——. "These Probiotics Lower Histamine (Rather Than Raising It)." Healing Histamine. https://healinghistamine.com/these-probiotic-strains-lower-histamine-rather-than-raising-it.

ACKNOWLEDGMENTS

TO MY READERS

Thank you for trusting me to help you on your health journey. Your stories inspire me to do what I do, and I am so grateful to assist in your recovery. I will keep striving to learn and teach more so that I can help as many of you as I can.

TO MY FAMILY

Jake, Levi and Liam, you are the beautiful boys that motivate me to be the best person I can be every day. You are my biggest supporters and I couldn't do half of what I do without you. I love you!

To my mom, Nannette, you are the strongest person I know and have taught me so much. Thank you for believing in me and helping me so that I am able to do all the things I do. You are the reason I have been able to put in the time needed to write these books.

To my sister, Naomi, and my dad, Steve, thank you for showing me the lighter side of life and reminding me to take time to laugh and have fun. I love you!

TO MY FRIENDS

Lynn Whitefall, you are my best friend and I am the luckiest person in the world to be in your life. You make me laugh every day and are always there when I need you. I love you so much!

Jennifer Robins, thank you for taking the time to help me when I had no idea what I was doing and for becoming one of my best friends in the process. You are such a giving person and I will always be grateful for you.

Brittney Bradway, thank you for all that you do for the Dr. Becky Campbell brand and for me in general. Your dedication to me and the patients in our practice is amazing, and I could not do any of this without you. Thank you also for being an amazing friend.

TO MY PUBLISHING TEAM

Thank you, Marissa and Will, for taking a chance on me when no one knew who I was and for letting me create my vision and put it on these pages exactly how I saw it. You and the rest of the team at Page Street—Karen, Meg, Nichole, Jill—are amazing. Thank you so much!

Libby Volgyes, thank you so much for making this book even more beautiful than I envisioned. You are truly amazing.

ABOUT THE **AUTHOR**

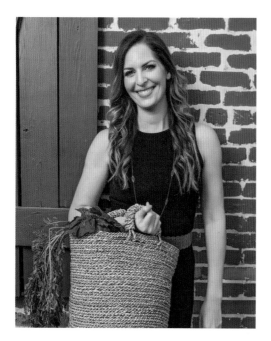

DR. BECKY CAMPBELL is a board-certified doctor of natural medicine who was initially introduced to functional medicine as a patient. She struggled with many of the issues her patients struggle with today, and she has made it her mission to help patients all around the world with her virtual practice. Dr. Becky Campbell is the founder of DrBeckyCampbell.com and author of *The 30-Day Thyroid Reset Plan*. She has been featured on multiple online publications like Mindbodygreen, Bustle, PopSugar and more. She has been a guest on many podcasts as a thyroid health and histamine intolerance expert. Dr. Campbell specializes in thyroid disease, autoimmune disease and histamine intolerance and hopes to help others regain their life as functional medicine helped her regain hers.

WORKING **WITH ME**

Are you ready to get the testing you need and start a protocol designed just for you? Many clients come to me when they want to get to the bottom of what may be going on. Here are some other reasons patients choose to work with a functional medicine practitioner:

- You don't want to rely on unnecessary drugs and medical intervention for the rest of your life.
- You are interested in discovering the underlying cause of your problems, rather than just suppressing your symptoms.
- You are motivated to play an active role in your own healing process.
- You are willing to make the necessary dietary and lifestyle changes to support health and well-being.

HOW DO I WORK WITH PATIENTS?

One way to think of functional medicine practitioners is as health detectives. We focus on identifying and addressing the underlying cause of an illness, rather than just suppressing symptoms.

Like all detectives, we use a variety of tools in our investigations, including detailed questionnaires, a thorough medical history and examination and comprehensive laboratory tests (blood, urine, stool, breath, hair testing and more).

We then use nutritional therapy, herbal medicine, supplements, stress management, detoxification, lifestyle changes and—in some cases and only when necessary—prescription medications to eliminate triggers and restore proper function and balance.

Deep and lasting healing is only possible when the root causes of illness are addressed. By understanding the core systems of the body, how they are related and how their function can be restored, many chronic illnesses can be prevented and even reversed.

WHAT IS MY TREATMENT PHILOSOPHY?

I practice a new model of medicine, sometimes referred to as functional or systems medicine. Functional medicine is neither conventional nor alternative medicine. It's a combination of the best elements of both, and it represents the future of medicine.

WHAT CONDITIONS DO I SPECIALIZE IN?

I have particular experience with and training in:

- Histamine intolerance
- Digestive problems and food intolerances
- Thyroid conditions
- Low immune function, allergies, asthma
- Autoimmune diseases
- Hormone imbalances (adrenal, thyroid, sex hormones)
- High cholesterol
- Fatigue, low energy, poor sleep
- Cognitive and neurological disorders

If you're ready to get started, contact me at https://DrBeckyCampbell.com.

INDEX